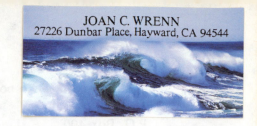

Medical Choice
in a Mexican Village

James Clay Young
Linda C. Garro

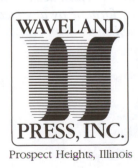

WAVELAND
PRESS, INC.

Prospect Heights, Illinois

For information about this book, write or call:

Waveland Press, Inc.
P.O. Box 400
Prospect Heights, Illinois 60070
(708) 634-0081

The cover photograph depicts an episode described on page 110 of this book involving Doña Juana, a well-known local curer, and Lupe, a young girl suffering stomach problems. The curer is applying a second application of a herbal remedy to Lupe's stomach. Doña Juana continues an active practice despite severe arthritis that has deformed her hands.

Contents

List of Figures

List of Tables

vi

Preface, 1994

The relationship between what people think and what they do is explored in this study of medical decision making in a Mexican village. It was motivated by the observation that in cultural settings characterized by multiple treatment options, there is significant variability in resort to different treatment alternatives by individuals and within families. How can this variability be explained? What considerations do individuals perceive as important? Are there shared cultural understandings which help account for different treatment decisions?

This book documents our attempt to answer these questions within the context of a single community. Central to the methodological design is a separation between the data used to build the decision model and that used to test the model. In addition to traditional ethnographic means, a variety of structured data collection methods are used. Detailed descriptions of the interviews, analysis and interpretation are provided in order to clarify the steps involved in independently building and testing the decision model.

It is not necessary, nor may it be culturally appropriate, for researchers attempting to assess the generalizability of our findings to faithfully replicate the specific interview procedures. The strategies used to elicit and construct decision models will vary by cultural context. What is critical is that efforts to assess the generalizability of the decision modeling approach be based on a two-pronged design which replicates the separation of data used in the construction of the model from data used in evaluation. Although we think that aspects of the findings have application to other settings which share similar characteristics, this can only be established through additional empirical work. The decision model developed here is not intended to pertain to any cultural setting but is tied to a particular ethnographic context. The findings of the present study cannot be invalidated simply by demonstrating that the model developed here does not fit another setting.

The cognitive anthropological approach adopted here focuses on representing the cultural understandings relevant to treatment decisions. But framing this study around the concept of choice may be seen by some as problematic. Choice is seen as implying that individuals are free to make voluntary decisions; it also minimizes attention to constraints imposed by political economy and the objective social order. Yet, such a critique begs the question of whether it is possible to explain what people do when faced with an illness, and why they do it, without recourse to cultural understandings. In addition, empirical studies of treatment choice have not been carried out from a political economy perspective. Such an account would have to explain why individuals resort to different alternatives at different times. Finally, it is incorrect to view an ethnographic decision model as fundamentally volitional. The model specifies only those alternatives that individuals in a cultural setting view as open to them. While a treatment alternative may be preferred, the model also stipulates the constraints that lead to the use of less preferred alternatives. These statements should not be interpreted as suggesting that a political economy perspective would not contribute to our understanding of treatment choice in Pichataro. On the contrary, each approach could be used to complement the other. They are not mutually exclusive.

In addition to accounting for treatment choices, a decision model can be evaluated in terms of its representation of the cognitive basis of decisions. Recent work in cognitive anthropology has emphasized the importance of goals to an understanding of human action. Although the formulation of the decision model in this book does not refer to goals, it is worthwhile to reconceptualize the findings in these terms.

Integral to the decision rules are two inverse rank orderings of treatment alternatives, a cost ordering and a probability-of-cure ordering. When an illness is not serious, the general pattern is to use the treatment alternatives in order of their costs, from least expensive to most expensive, as a last resort. When the illness is judged to be serious, the preferred pattern is to use the alternative most likely to result in a cure, with cost a much less important consideration. Although both of these orderings are based on a general goal of getting well, embedded in cost-ordering is the goal of conserving economic resources and within the probability-of-cure ordering, the goal of ensuring that a cure is achieved. In the decision process these goals may conflict as physician treatment is generally the alternative judged most likely to achieve a cure but is also the most expensive, while self-treatment is judged least likely to achieve a cure and is also the least expensive. These goals are prioritized on the basis of illness severity. In the probability-of-cure ordering priority is placed on obtaining an efficacious cure. In the cost-ordered strategy, the emphasis is on spending as little as possible to achieve a cure.

The two orderings represent prototypical patterns and, of course, there are exceptions, especially when the means are not available to realize a particular choice. For example, when a serious illness occurs in a household with scarce economic resources, even though the preferred choice would be the alternative with the highest likelihood of cure, economic limitations constrain choices to lower costs, thereby approximating a cost-ordered sequence. The decision model consists of rules which incorporate these general principles of preferred sources of treatment and details the constraints that at times lead to the choice of less preferred alternatives. These rules should not be reified as constructs in people's heads, but are generated in response to particular illness situations and operative constraints. While the two orderings represent the goals people have in mind when making treatment decisions, whether these goals are realized depends in part on the presence or absence of external constraints such as lack of money or transportation.

This book now bears the names of both of the individuals responsible for its creation. Before this book was first published, my late husband asked to have my name added as an author. He was told it was too late in the process to make this change as well as other changes that would be required (e.g., the consistent use of ''we'' throughout the text). At the time, I was pursuing a graduate degree in another field and considered the omission unimportant. Subsequently, the loss of my husband and the realization of the depth of my interest in anthropological problems, led to a major career shift. The decision to add my name was a difficult one, but only because of concern about possible negative reactions by others. However, when a book represents the joint work of two individuals it cannot be inappropriate for that fact to be reflected by joint authorship which recognizes the primary role of the senior author. Nevertheless, changes have not been introduced into the text that is reprinted here in its original form.

—Linda C. Garro

Preface

This study of medical beliefs and illness treatment decision making is based on field research done in collaboration with my wife, Linda C. Garro. It employs what we regard as one of the more promising contemporary anthropological methods—the cognitive-ethnographic study of decision making in natural settings. Our aim has been to use this approach in investigating medical choice in Pichátaro, a village in the mountains of west-central Mexico, in such a way that the findings will be of interest not only to anthropologists, but to anyone concerned with how people in rural Third World communities deal with the universal problem of illness. *Medical Choice in a Mexican Village* is my account of the results of these efforts.

In the course of the research we have incurred many debts, which I would like to acknowledge here. Thanks must go first to the people of Pichátaro, who responded to our presence in their community—and to our unending questions—with friendship and cooperation. I cannot begin to name all who served as our willing teachers, but there are some I must thank individually. I offer sincere appreciation to Octavio, Francisco, and Rafael Equihua for the many hours spent in their company. We were also warmly received in our innumerable visits to the homes of Mateo Rodriguez and Martín and Rogelio Martinez, and they have my heartfelt thanks. I owe much to Rafael Espinosa for his incisive and eloquent views on life in Pichátaro.

Dr. Gonzalo Aguirre Beltrán of the Secretaría de Educación Pública, and Gildardo Gonzalez Ramos and Alberto Medina Pérez of the Instituto Nacional Indigenista, provided valuable advice and assistance. The Instituto Nacional de Antropología e Historia, and its subdirector, Fernando Cámara Barbachano, have my thanks for their cooperation in granting permission for the field research.

At the Department of Anthropology of the University of California, Riverside, where I received my training in anthropology, I would especially like to acknowledge the advice and help of Alan Beals, David Kronenfeld, Michael Kearney, Gene Anderson, Carol Mukhopadhyay, and Robert Randall. Others who have contributed to the project, both with their advice and with the examples they have set in their own work, include Christina Gladwin, Hugh Gladwin, and Naomi Quinn. Of course, none of these people should be held responsible for any shortcomings remaining in this work.

John Maiolo and Walter Shepherd of East Carolina University provided valuable support during final revision of the manuscript, for which they have my thanks. Those who assisted with the preparation of the manuscript include Karen DeVol and Shirley Lassiter, who typed the final version, Joan Mansfield, who produced several of the figures, and Ellen Schrader and Bonnie Ratcliff, who assisted with the index. I appreciate the efforts of Marlie Wasserman and Leslie Mitchner of Rutgers University Press, who saw the manuscript through the publication process with skill and care.

The research was funded by a grant-in-aid from the Wenner-Gren Foundation for Anthropological Research, and by Alcohol, Drug Abuse, and Mental Health Administration National Research Service Awards Nos. 1–F31–MH–05500–01 and 5–F31–MH–05500–02 from the National Institute of Mental Health. I am pleased to acknowledge this generous support.

Chapter Four was previously published, in slightly different form, as "Illness Categories and Action Strategies in a Tarascan Town" in *American Ethnologist* (5:1:1978:81–97, copyright American Anthropological Association), and is used here with permission. It is again my pleasure to acknowledge the advice of James Armstrong in that analysis. Portions of Chapter Six appeared in somewhat different form in my article "A Model of Illness Treatment Decisions in a Tarascan Town" in *American Ethnologist* (7:1:1980: 106–131).

Spanish terms have been used in the text wherever they add precision to the ethnographic description; those used repeatedly are defined in the Glossary.

To protect the privacy of our informants, the names used in the text have been changed.

Our initial fieldwork was carried out during twelve months' residence in Pichátaro from 1975 to 1977. We spent several more weeks there doing further field research in the summer of 1980. The pattern of use of different health-care alternatives remains basically as described here. The formal model of treatment decision making presented in Chapter Six would seem fully as adequate for these more recent data as for the 1975–1977 cases. We also had the opportunity to collect data in the neighboring community of Uricho, which has better access to Western health care. This will allow us to begin exploring the wider applicability of the conclusions reached in Chapter Seven.

I would again like to acknowledge the contributions of my wife, Linda, to this project. She did as much of the interviewing as I. Her continuing advice and assistance as I analyzed the data and wrote up the findings have been essential to the completion of this book. Whatever merit it has is as much due to her efforts as to my own, and for this she has my most sincere thanks of all.

Medical Choice
in a Mexican Village

1

Introduction

This is an anthropological study of a rural Mexican community's system of medical beliefs, and of how these beliefs relate to the way people deal with illness. The focus of the study is on individuals as purposive actors and rational decision makers. We attempt to understand the nature of the knowledge they bring to an occurrence of illness, how this knowledge is applied in evaluating the illness, and the process whereby decisions about treatment are then made. The setting is a village having a pluralistic health-care system, in which orthodox Western medical care is only one of several alternative sources of treatment.

The situation examined here is by no means unique. People everywhere must choose from the several possible courses of action available to them in attempting to treat illness. The question of choice becomes even more significant in non-Western settings, where modern medical services, often only recently having become available, represent alternatives to longer-established traditional medical practices and native curing specialists.[1] This kind of medical pluralism is common in countries of the Third World, particularly in their rural communities. People in these settings have an especially varied set of options and must regularly choose from among two or more distinct systems of medical knowledge and practice in seeking treatment for an illness. The present study attempts, in the context of one such community, to explain how these choices are made.

This explanation is based on a formal model of the decision-making process employed by members of the community in seeking treatment. The model is constructed within the framework of recent developments in cognitive anthropology concerning decision making in natural, real-world situations. Studies of this type have attempted to move from the earlier ethnoscience concern with the

3

content and organization of particular domains of cultural knowledge (see Tyler 1969) to the question of how such knowledge relates
to purposive behavior by describing the shared decision rules by
which people select alternative actions. Thus we are concerned not
only with what a people believes to be true about illness and its
treatment but also with the specific consequences of these beliefs
for what they do about illness.

THE STUDY OF MEDICAL CHOICE

One of the best ways to examine how alternative medical systems
interrelate is from the point of view of the people who must choose
among them. Much of the existing research by anthropologists interested in illness beliefs and treatment practices has in fact dealt
with the issue of choice, although with a variety of purposes and
from several theoretical-methodological perspectives.[2] Implicit in
these differing approaches to medical choice are somewhat differing
views of what constitutes explanation.

Crucial to understanding the aims of the present research, in contrast to these others, is the distinction between culture as patterned
events and behavior and culture as a system of knowledge. Both of
these are current views of what culture is or represents (for example, contrast Harris 1968 and Kay 1970). But as Goodenough (1964)
has pointed out, these are not merely two differing views of the
same reality; they point to two distinct orders of reality:

> One is the phenomenal order of observed events and the regulari-
> ties they exhibit. A human community, like any other natural uni-
> verse in a state of near equilibrium, exhibits the statistical patterns
> characteristic of internally stable systems. . . . Similar, but never
> identical, events occur over and over again and are therefore isolable
> as types of event and patterned arrangement. Certain types of ar-
> rangement tend to persist and others to appear and reappear in fixed
> sequences. An observer can perceive this kind of statistical pattern-
> ing in a community without any knowledge whatever of the ideas,
> beliefs, values, and principles of action of the community's members,
> the ideational order. The phenomenal order is a property of the com-
> munity as a material system of people, their surroundings, and their

behavior. The ideational order is a property not of the community
but of its members. It is their organization of their experience within
the phenomenal order, a product of cognitive and instrumental
(habit forming) learning. The ideational order, unlike the statistical
order, is nonmaterial, being composed of ideal forms as they exist in
people's minds, propositions about their interrelationships, preference ratings regarding them, and recipes for their mutual ordering as
means to desired ends. . . . Thus, the phenomenal order of a community, its characteristic "way of life," is an artifact of the ideational
order of its members (Goodenough 1964:11–12).

Culture, in the sense of the ideational order, provides the people of
a community with, among other things, shared standards or rules
for solving problems and selecting particular courses of action. Of
course, a cultural tradition cannot provide reliable standards for
behavior in all possible situations. But, in general, the more recurrent and important the choice, the more likely it is that we will be
able to elicit meaningful statements of how these choices are made
(Quinn 1978:220). Illness would seem to fit these qualifications, and
thus we will assume that the best way of explaining the observable
pattern of illness treatment choices characterizing a community is
to discover, in as direct a way as possible, the ideational basis of
these choices in the minds of the community's members.

Thus we advocate that systematic attention be given to people's
own explanations of the considerations they have in mind in their
choices of treatment. In contrast, much other research on medical
choice in pluralistic settings either explicitly rejects the formal elic-
itation of decision criteria as a major research strategy or more frequently, implicitly eliminates it with the adoption of a correlational paradigm. A good example of explicit rejection is Janzen's
(1978) study of therapeutic choices among the BaKongo of Lower
Zaire. That study analyzes a small number of especially complex
illnesses in the belief that such cases would best clarify the multiple
relationships between alternative treatments and the ways in
which the actors evaluate their options. Janzen follows particular
cases through time and interprets the resulting therapeutic choices
on the basis of informants' post hoc "rationalizations," combined
with his knowledge of the particular social position and personal

history of the patient. He specifically contrasts this approach with that in which people are asked, in formal interviews, to explain the nature of the considerations involved in their decisions about treatment. Janzen's attempt to employ this latter approach, which he identifies with ethnoscience, was reported to have been unsuccessful—it resulted only in "cerebralized and individualized reconstructions of native theory" (1978:34)—and was thus discarded.[3] Since it is just this kind of approach that is followed here, it is important to clarify the probable reasons for Janzen's difficulties.

Janzen's main problem seems related to the nature of his cases. By specifically concentrating on those that were unusually complex, problematic, and that had escalated beyond the ordinary (1978:64), he minimized the likelihood that such routine decision-making standards, as described above, would be operative. The decisions he considers were undoubtedly of great importance to the people involved, but because all ordinary means to cope with them failed, they were inherently less predictable. Thus Janzen's attempts to discover culturally standardized decision rules would understandably be inconclusive. In fact, anthropologists looking at therapeutic choice in pluralistic settings have often tended to concentrate on the unusual and the spectacular at the expense of the more mundane, but much more frequent—and in the long term more significant—kinds of illnesses people deal with in daily life. To be sure, examination of extraordinary cases can yield significant insights into the dynamics of medical pluralism, but to concentrate exclusively on such nonroutine decision making leaves us largely unprepared to account for how most of a group's members make decisions about treating most kinds of illnesses most of the time. It is just this sort of an accounting that the present study attempts to accomplish.

In contrast to the "thick description" (see Geertz 1973) approach of Janzen, Turner (1968), and others, a large number of studies of medical choice have adopted what I referred to as a "correlational" paradigm. In this approach, single factors or variables, or classes of these, are posited as explaining aggregate data on differential treatment choices because of their patterns of association with them. Studies done within this framework, for the most part, may be classified according to whether they have emphasized either characteristics of the illnesses tending to be taken to each treatment alternative, or characteristics of the people tending to use each alternative. For example, in some Latin American communities it has been reported (see Erasmus 1952; G. Foster 1958; Simmons 1955) that illnesses are generally classified into two groups: those that are curable with modern medicine, and those that can be successfully treated only with folk curing methods. Treatment choices, in this view, then become predictable on the basis of the diagnostic category of the particular episode, and its status relative to this "folk dichotomy." [4] Alternatively, several studies (see DeWalt 1977; McClain 1977; Press 1969; Schwartz 1969; Woods 1977; Woods and Graves 1973) have focused primarily on the characteristics of the people tending to use different treatment sources. These studies assert that some people in a community use different treatment alternatives because they have different beliefs or expectations about their effectiveness. Accordingly, individual characteristics such as educational level, acculturative status, age, and sex would seem likely to show significant relationships with treatment choices. Studies of this type base their explanation on the discovery of co-occurring phenomena, with the implicit assertion that there is some necessity to this co-occurrence, some sort of causal connection. This assertion has been suitably criticized elsewhere (see, for example, Fisher and Werner 1978:206). As a means of providing a truly cultural explanation of medical choice, the correlational approach poses a number of difficulties.

A common misconception is that choice of treatment involves only two alternatives—traditional and modern medicine. While this is a distinction that the investigator may well wish to make in the course of analysis, it does not necessarily represent the only, or even the most salient, distinction among treatment alternatives in the minds of the people making the choices. In most settings described—and this is certainly also true in the present case—there are multiple sources of both modern and traditional medical treatment. It is necessary not only to recognize that in most settings there exist several major alternatives, including self-treatment, but also to take care that these alternatives represent the entire range of options in the view of the people being studied as well.

Another difficulty is that studies of this type sometimes lack extensive data to support their conclusions, and base broad generalizations on relatively few cases. It is revealing, for example, that at least in the case of the community studied here, illness types which clearly fit into the type of folk dichotomy described earlier represent considerably less than 10% of all illness episodes recorded. A related consideration in associating certain diagnostic categories with specific alternatives is that the label applied to a given illness episode by an informant, particularly if questioned some time after the illness has occurred, is often not independent of the treatment chosen.

The most fundamental criticism to be made of the correlational approach, however, is that in looking primarily at overall patterns of treatment choices and their regularities in terms of the type of illness or class of people associated with each alternative, the ideational basis of the many individual decisions these patterns ultimately represent is largely ignored or, at best, is only indirectly inferred. And since varied considerations may lead to the same observable outcome, or conversely, a variety of actions may be taken by different people applying basically the same standards of choice, investigations that deal primarily with the phenomenal order can inform us only imprecisely, and often incorrectly, about the ideational basis of the observed behavior. This is not to say that the phenomenal order may be ignored. To the contrary, the actual, observable outcomes associated with different occurrences of illness will be precisely the data used to verify our description of the ideational basis of these choices.

With only a few exceptions (see A. Beals 1976; Fabrega 1974), research on choices of treatment in pluralistic settings has thus not been primarily concerned with discovering and explicitly modeling the decision-making process. This study will attempt to show the advantages of this method of inquiry.

THE DECISION-MAKING APPROACH

Although the idea that anthropologists should concern themselves with individual decision making is not a particularly new one (see Firth 1951; Goodenough 1956; Barth 1967), only relatively recently, as part of the growth of the field of cognitive ethnography, have explicit methodologies for undertaking such studies been developed (see Geoghegan 1973; C. Gladwin 1977; Kay 1970; Quinn 1974). My purpose is not to review these developments (for such reviews, see Quinn 1975; White 1973) but instead briefly to outline what studies emphasizing the decision-making approach represent and what they attempt to accomplish.

Anthropologists employing this perspective have generally assumed that in areas of life in which people must regularly choose between alternative courses of action, the members of a given group frequently come to have a common set of standards concerning how such choices are made. To the extent that members share similar relevant beliefs and purposes, and similar means for realizing these purposes, and also have available similar alternative courses of action, the idea of shared standards of choice seems justified. A decision model represents an attempt to describe these standards in an explicit, precise, and testable manner. Thus far, although the number of empirical applications of the approach is small, the results obtained have generally been quite good: usually 80% or more of the choices are correctly accounted for (see H. Gladwin et al. 1978; Kay 1970).

A decision-making study usually addresses three questions (see C. Gladwin 1977; Quinn 1976): 1. What are the alternatives the members of a group consider open to them in regard to the particular problem at hand? 2. What are the criteria they use in selecting among these alternatives (what information is considered)? 3. What is the decision process—the principles whereby this information is used or manipulated in making a choice? These findings may then be formalized in a model (such as a flow chart, decision tree, or decision table) that specifies the different ways in which specific considerations or states of relevant criteria lead to the choice of each alternative. Once constructed, the model may be tested using independent data on the actual choices made by members of the study community in selecting from among these alternatives. The extent to which the model is found to account correctly for the observed choices then serves as the measure of its accuracy in depicting the actual standards of choice involved.[5]

Ethnographic models of decision-making processes constitute an alternative to models which, for purposes of formal elegance, attribute to the decision maker complex calculations of the overall benefits or utilities associated with each alternative. A number of recent studies (Fjellman 1976; C. Gladwin 1976, 1977; Quinn 1976; Tversky 1972) would argue that models of decision making that do entail such calculations are cognitively unrealistic in terms of the information processing capabilities they would require, and because of this cannot offer accurate representations of everyday choice making. Instead, it is argued, people are able to make complex decisions by relying on procedures which simplify the kinds of cognitive operations required; a major research aim is to discover the process whereby this simplification is accomplished. One consequence of simplification is that optimal choices—those having highest utility, lowest costs, or greatest benefits—are not always, and probably not even routinely, made (Simon 1957). Because of this, outcomes in natural decision making are determined both by the nature of the information considered and by the nature of how it is processed. Following Quinn (1976, 1978), then, we may assume that models which come closest to representing real-world decision processes should also generate the most accurate predictions of behavior. Thus it becomes essential that the procedures used in the construction of such models entail no presumptions about the ultimate form of the process itself.

THE FIELD RESEARCH

The analysis of medical choice presented in this book is based on materials collected in Pichátaro, Michoacán, a rural community in west-central Mexico. My wife and I were full-time residents of the town from October 1975 to August 1976, and subsequently from June to August of 1977, for a period totaling just over twelve months. All interviewing, which with very few exceptions was done in Spanish (Pichátaro is a bilingual community),[6] as well as other data collection, were carried out either by myself or my wife, a psychologist with considerable anthropological training. Our informants included members of probably one-fifth of the over five hundred households in town. A smaller number, perhaps twenty-five or thirty, we came to know well, and it is from these people that we acquired the bulk of our education in Pichátaro's culture.

Most of the formally collected data may be placed in one of three categories: 1. data used in developing the model of treatment choice; 2. data used in testing the model; and 3. background and supporting data. A brief review of the procedures employed in each of these areas may serve to illustrate the overall plan of the fieldwork. Each of the interviewing methods is described in greater detail later in the book.

The data used in developing the model of treatment choice are from a series of interviews that constituted one of the main fieldwork activities during almost eight months of our residence. These interviews, which were done with a core group of approximately fifteen informants, were aimed at eliciting data on both the decision criteria and the decision process. All except the initial interviews (the "paired comparisons," described in Chapter Six) involved procedures that were devised or extensively modified in the field in response to data needs that became apparent as the research progressed. In all, we completed five different kinds of interviews, each directed at a specific aspect of the choice process.

Once the interviewing for the decision model was under way, we began concurrent work on collecting case history materials for eventual use in testing the model. For a period of about six months, from February to late July 1976, a representative sample of sixty-two Pichátaro households was surveyed on an approximate biweekly basis. At each visit, detailed descriptions of illnesses that had occurred in the household were recorded on a standardized form. None of the households involved in the interviewing described in the first category was included in the sample; the cases therefore provide independent data with which to test the model. In all, 323 illness episodes were recorded, providing a fairly extensive, varied, and generally representative view of the occurrence of illness in Pichátaro.[7] Background data on the households in the sample were also collected. For each, brief descriptions were obtained of past illnesses that had occurred prior to the case collection period. These household illness histories provided useful information on the kinds of illness known by a given family and its experiences with different treatment alternatives. These data were particularly important in making the actual test of the model, as is described in Chapter Six. We also collected fairly extensive socio-economic data on each of the households to determine the degree to which such factors may account for the different treatment choices (see Appendix B). Finally, several key informants were asked to rate the households in the sample in terms of their relative level of wealth. These ratings were used in assigning an overall wealth rank to each household. (Additional details on the case collection procedures and the wealth rankings are given in Appendix A.)

Throughout the research period, data were collected to provide background both for the study in general, and for the treatment decision model in particular. Early in the fieldwork we completed a census of Pichátaro's 509 households. This provided data on the town's population structure, the distribution of occupational types, language usage, household composition, educational levels, and so on. The census taking, along with a town mapping project that preceded it, also served to introduce us to the residents: by early in the research period, each household in town had been visited by at least one of us, and the general purpose of our presence in Pichátaro explained. The census materials supplemented our less formal observations as participants in many of the routine affairs of the town. We attended fiestas, masses, town meetings, weddings, and funerals, and questioned people about what we had seen. We made friends, became ritual kinsmen, got sick and were cured, engaged in town gossip, visited, and in general experienced town life to the extent that our position as obvious, but graciously accepted, outsiders permitted. Much of the description in the following chapter, in particular, derives from this sort of informal data collection.

People's decisions about treatment necessarily cannot be understood in isolation from their more general beliefs about illness. Accordingly, much of the interviewing not specifically involved with the development of the decision model dealt with a number of related aspects of Pichátaro's medical system—concepts of bodily structure and functioning, ideas about illness causation, principles of symptom evaluation, illness diagnosis and classification, and traditional treatment practices. A structured interview was designed to sample illness beliefs in terms of the attributes of a set of named illness types, and a formal analysis of the data it provided illustrates several features of Pichátaro's illness categories. Much effort was also directed at identifying and determining the features of the entire range of alternative sources of treatment used by Pichatareños. (Pichatareño refers to a person from, or a thing characteristic of, Pichátaro.) Practitioners of each type in the community were interviewed, and visits were made to nonlocal treatment facilities used by townspeople.

THE PLAN OF THE BOOK

Chapter Two describes the community of our research, with emphasis on those aspects of town life, and of the town's relation to the larger Mexican society, having greatest relevance for health care.

The focus then turns specifically to the Pichátaro medical system. Chapter Three introduces the main features of folk medical knowledge. It describes the basis of these beliefs in local conceptions of bodily structure and function, as well as the variety of principles invoked in explaining illness. Particular attention is given to the illness evaluation process and to the factors involved in judgments of seriousness—which are later shown to have special significance in the treatment decision process.

Chapter Four illustrates some of the linkages between this system of knowledge and the actions that people take in response to illness. A formal analysis of a sampling of illness beliefs shows that the structuring of illness categories tends to be congruent with how this knowledge is used in purposive action relating to illness. These findings challenge the relevance of etiological concepts such as the "hot"-"cold" system as determinants of some types of illness-related behavior.

The next two chapters directly address the issue of choice of treatment. Chapter Five describes the range of treatment alternatives used by town residents. Chapter Six presents the formal model of treatment decision making in Pichátaro, including details on the methods used in its construction and verification.

The concluding chapter summarizes the findings concerning the use of each of the principal treatment options and goes on to consider the major implications of the study for health care policy in pluralistic settings like that of Pichátaro. It demonstrates that some of the more accepted views on the factors limiting the use of modern medicine by rural Third World peoples do not adequately explain the situation in Pichátaro, and presents an alternative explanation.

2

Pichátaro, a Sierra
Tarascan Town

The decisions that the people of Pichátaro make in dealing with illness are in a very real way influenced by the particular conditions in which they live. The kinds of health hazards to which they are exposed, the options they have available in treating illness, and the constraints operating in choices among these are all determined by the nature of their community and its place in relation to the wider society. In this chapter we will examine Pichátaro, its people, and their ways of life, with special attention to those aspects most important for understanding the broader context of medical choice.[1]

THE REGION AND THE TOWN

San Francisco Pichátaro is a Tarascan community of nearly three thousand people located in the west-central Mexican state of Michoacán.[2] The town lies at an altitude of around 8,000 feet in the *tierra fría* ('cold country'), west of Lake Pátzcuaro, and is some twenty miles by road from the regional market city of Pátzcuaro (see Figure 2.1). This part of Michoacán divides into two main areas: the Sierra Tarasca, the largest, comprising the western two-thirds of the region; and the string of towns and villages around the shore and on the islands of Lake Pátzcuaro. The Sierra is a high volcanic plateau with an irregular surface of interlacing mountains and valleys, formed largely from composite volcanoes, lava flows, and younger cinder cones—one of which (Parícutin) appeared only forty years ago. Due to its elevation, the Sierra is an area of generally cool days and cold nights. The year divides into a wet season, with almost daily rain from late May or early June until Septem-

15

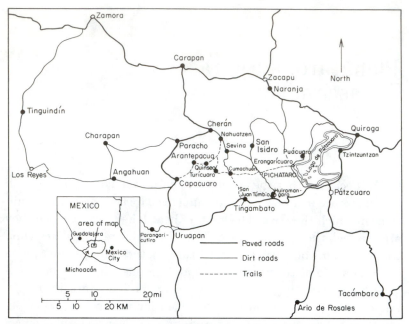

Figure 2.1.   **The Tarascan Area of Michoacán, Mexico**

ber, and a dry season of usually clear, but often windy and dusty days during the remaining months. Areas of the Sierra that have not long since been cleared for agriculture—such areas include almost all reasonably flat land—are covered with mixed pine and deciduous forests. To a North American eye the Sierra is an area of considerable natural beauty, with its crisp, clear air, sometimes brilliantly blue skies, lush green countryside, and cool forests. Scattered through the Sierra are over forty towns *(pueblos)* and an even greater number of smaller settlements or *ranchos,* usually located on level ground near natural sources of water. The economy of most Sierra towns depends upon agriculture, primarily but not exclusively the cultivation of maize. To varying degrees farming is supplemented with handicraft production and the exploitation of forest resources. Bordering the eastern edge of the Sierra, and around 1,000 feet lower in elevation, is the Lake district, an area of gentler slopes reaching down to the shores of shallow, crescent-shaped Lake Pátzcuaro. The Lake area generally enjoys a milder

climate than the Sierra, although sharing with it the same pattern
of wet and dry seasons. Vegetation here is more sparse, and pines
are notably absent. Around the Lake are located some twenty
pueblos and numerous ranchos, including several located on islands
in the lake itself.[3]

Tarascan, or *porépecha* as it is called in that tongue, is an American Indian language spoken by about fifty thousand persons (Friedrich 1976) currently living in the area included in Figure 2.1. The
majority of these are bilingual Tarascan-Spanish speakers; at most,
monolinguals represent but 20% of the total (M. Foster 1969; Mexico 1963; see also West 1948:20). The linguistic affiliation of Tarascan has never been clear, and despite some assertions of remote
connections to Zuñi and Quechua (see Swadesh 1969), no close ge-
netic relationship has yet been demonstrated (Friedrich 1970:9n;
M. Foster 1969).

The modern Tarascan region represents only a small fraction of
the total area included within the Tarascan Empire of pre-
Conquest times. At the time of the arrival of the Spanish in the
mid-1500's, the area of Tarascan speech extended over most of the
present-day state of Michoacán, and into parts of Jalisco and Gue-
rrero; the political limits of their empire reached even further
(West 1948:11). The ancient Tarascans were notable for having
been one of the few groups adjacent to the Aztecs that never fell
under the latter's domination. The coming of the Spanish, however,
was generally disastrous for the Tarascans, who underwent a sharp
decrease in number, concomitant with the beginning of a recession
of the area of native speech that continued steadily over the next
few centuries, until all that remained was the nuclear area centered
in the Sierra and around Lake Pátzcuaro. Today the Tarascan area
is one of Mexico's several "regions of refuge" (Aguirre Beltrán
1967)—relatively isolated regions consisting of a hinterland of
largely Indian communities linked to a regional administrative and
market center. Such areas have in recent years been the foci of operations for several development programs and agencies of the
Mexican government.

Towns in the Tarascan area are generally identifiable as either
Indian or mestizo, based primarily on the extent to which the in-

digenous language is spoken. The existence of most Indian towns may be traced to pre-Conquest times. Mestizo towns represent either more recent settlements established by non-Tarascan-speaking immigrants to the area, or else formerly Indian towns in which Tarascan has long since ceased to be spoken. Those in the latter case tend to be, or to have been, important trade centers.[4]

The community of Pichátaro lies near the boundary separating the Sierra from the lake area. Although definitely a Sierra town, historically it has had important economic ties with the lake town of Erongarícuaro and the city of Pátzcuaro, the latter having even greater significance today. Pichátaro is situated in a long valley enclosed on three sides by pine-forested mountains. The floor of the valley is relatively flat, and almost entirely covered with fields. At present one enters town via a seven-mile stretch of dirt road that branches off from the Pátzcuaro-Uruapan highway near the towns of Huiramangaro and San Juan Túmbio. The road continues on from Pichátaro, passing through Sevina and Nahuatzen before joining the Carapan-Uruapan highway at Cherán (Figure 2.1). The construction of the road in 1971–1972 had important consequences for life in Pichátaro, an issue which will be taken up in more detail later.

The town is laid out in the Spanish grid pattern, having quite uniform blocks in its central part but becoming more irregular as one goes toward the outskirts (see Figure 2.2). Along its dirt and cobbled streets are collected slightly over five hundred individual household compounds. The settlement is compact, with interspersed corn fields occurring only occasionally on the edges of town. The center of Pichátaro is the area around the plaza, where one finds the offices of the town government, one of the two primary schools, the medical post, the civil registry, the new secondary school, the potable water office, the town's only telephone, and, immediately to the south, the church and convent.

One thing that would likely impress a visitor to Pichátaro, particularly one who ventured from the main street, are the handsome and solidly built wood plank houses *(trojes)* characteristic of the Tarascan Sierra. A typical household compound includes a *troje* and two or three less substantial buildings, enclosed with a piled

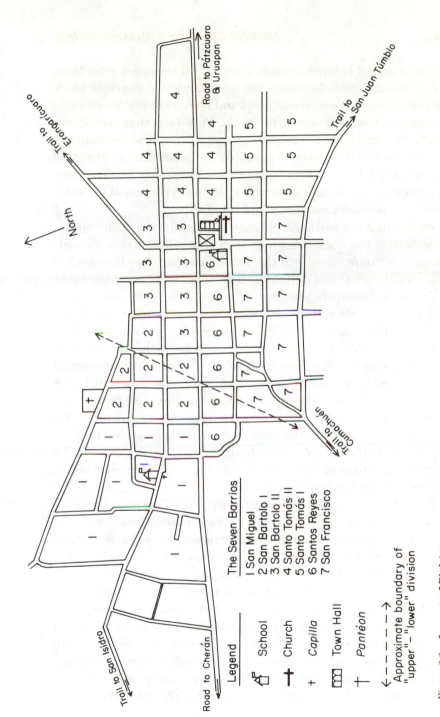

The Seven Barrios
1 San Miguel
2 San Bartolo I
3 San Bartolo II
4 Santo Tomás II
5 Santo Tomás I
6 Santos Reyes
7 San Francisco

Legend

School

Church

+ Capilla

Town Hall

+ Pantéon

Approximate boundary of
"upper"–"lower" division

North

Trail to Erongarícuaro

Road to Pátzcuaro & Uruapan

Trail to San Juan Túmblo

Trail to Cumachuén

Trail to San Isidro

Road to Cherán

Figure 2.2. Layout of Pichátaro

stone fence and entered through a heavy, shake-roofed gate. More recent construction, however, has been largely of concrete block and brick due to the increasing cost and scarcity of lumber suitable for *trojes*. A second aspect of life in Pichátaro that would undoubtedly catch the visitor's attention are the inescapable *tocadiscos*—record players connected to loudspeakers that are hoisted atop tall poles, broadcasting their music over large sections of town. As many as half a dozen may be heard playing at the same time, each set at an ear-shattering volume.

Pichátaro is not particularly large—it takes about fifteen minutes to walk from one end to the other. Its high population density leads the outsider unfamiliar with this fact to assume that the town has fewer inhabitants than it actually does. The tight concentration of homes rather abruptly gives way to maize fields on the north, east, and west sides of town. To the south one walks first through the orchards, for which Pichátaro is regionally famous, and then reaches the fields. Beyond these in most directions one then encounters wooded mountains, still part of Pichátaro's lands, which are exploited for firewood, lumber, and pine resin—the last being an important source of extra cash for many families. Also to be found here are several springs, one of which supplies the town's piped water system. Apart from the road, several trails, passable by foot, burro, or horse, radiate out from Pichátaro leading to the neighboring towns of Cumachuén, San Juan Túmbio, San Isidro, Sevina, and Erongarícuaro.

Pichátaro has undoubtedly existed since pre-Conquest times, although neither with its present settlement pattern nor possibly in its present location. The *Relación de Michoacán,* an early colonial document compiled around 1540 that provides some insight into pre-Conquest Tarascan society, makes passing mention of "Pechataro." It is first described as a hunting place of the Tarascan lords, and brief note is later made of the lord Ypinchuani who, along with his god Tiripenie Xugapeti, established himself here (Craine and Reindorp 1970:110,112). A local legend recounts how Pichátaro once consisted of seven separate villages, "each with its own king." Only one of these, Chátaru (from where the town's name is said to have come), was located at the modern site. The other six are said to have been scattered in the hills around Pichátaro. At some point a very long time ago these seven came together and created one village, each of the former units retaining its identity as one of the seven *barrios* of present-day Pichátaro. This account seems quite plausible in view of the sixteenth-century Spanish policy of concentrating Indians living in scattered settlements into more easily administered units (Hunt and Nash 1967:260). Other evidence of the town's antiquity is provided by the poorly preserved archaeological remains of what appears to have been a small stone platform, south of town, and by the small ceramic figures occasionally unearthed by Pichátaro farmers while plowing their fields.

THE PEOPLE OF PICHATARO

In the Tarascan area (as elsewhere in Mexico) there was in the past a distinction made between *gente natural* ('natural people') and *gente de razón* ('people of reason'), the former referring to the Tarascan-speaking people native to the area, the latter to the Spanish-speaking mestizo population. Today one hears these terms used only by older Pichatareños, most others rightly resenting the implication that they are somehow without reason, and preferring to refer to themselves as *gente indígena* ('indigenous people'). As in Mesoamerica generally, the features distinguishing an Indian from a mestizo have less to do with actual biological characteristics (both may be considerably "mixed" from this point of view), than with cultural characteristics such as dress and especially language. Well over 90% of the people in Pichátaro may be identified, and indeed would identify themselves, as Indian (although not all of these speak Tarascan). Traditionally, stores in Pichátaro were run primarily by mestizo families from Spanish-speaking towns in the area, but today this is less the case.

Ethnic relations in the Tarascan area have little of the castelike quality evident in some other areas of Mesoamerica, notably Chiapas and highland Guatemala. In everyday town life it is fair to say that the Indian-mestizo distinction has minimal significance in ordering interpersonal relations. When Pichatareños go to Pátzcuaro and other cities, however, they are likely to be addressed using the familiar *tú* form, to be spoken to with less courtesy in stores, and forced to wait longer before being attended. This is particularly true of women, who dress more traditionally than men, and hence are more readily identifiable as Indian. In their own theory of ethnic group differences, many local people view *gente indígena* such as themselves as physically superior to mestizos—as stronger, more resistant to illness, and more capable of bearing hardship and pain. The outside observer with a machismo, or aggressive manliness, stereotype of the Mexican male would find that it poorly characterizes the majority of Pichátaro men. Instead, one would likely be impressed with the average Pichatareño's reserve, great concern with etiquette, and painstaking avoidance of verbal offense, particularly when dealing with outsiders.

Our census of the community, completed early in 1976, showed a total population of just under 2,900 individuals. As shown in Figure 2.3, this is a young population—over 30% are under ten years of age, 44% are less than fifteen, and over half (55%) are under twenty. Pichátaro, like many rural Third World communities, clearly has a high growth potential, increasingly so as the mortality rate (now somewhat above the Mexican national rate) continues to decline in relation to a higher fertility rate. Pichátaro also has a high dependency ratio (the ratio of the population either too old or too young to work, to the population of working age). If we define the economically active producers as that segment of the population between ages fifteen and sixty-five, they are by a slight margin outnumbered by consumers (the segment of the population outside of this range)—a situation that on a national basis represents a high ratio indeed (see Matras 1973:51–52). This imbalance, combined with the relatively low productivity of a traditional subsistence technology, must be one of the more important constraints on increases in the overall level of living in the town.

Pichátaro is a bilingual community. The majority of persons older than about thirty or thirty-five learned Tarascan as their first language, and began to acquire Spanish at some later time. One informant described the time before he knew Spanish.

Rafael said that it was not until the coming of the movie house, the radio, and the *tocadiscos,* in the 1950's, that people began to learn

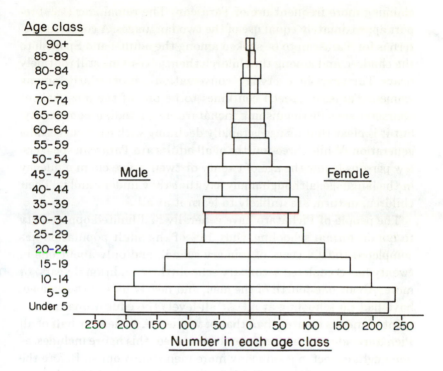

Figure 2.3. **Population Pyramid for Pichátaro—1976**

Spanish. Before that everyone spoke just Tarascan. In these times it was difficult to go to Pátzcuaro or Erongarícuaro and deal with the *gente de razón* even if you really needed something, like medicine. When he had to go, he would lay awake the night before, with his heart pounding, thinking "How, how am I going to tell them what I need?"

Increasing contact with outsiders, particularly in commerce, along with more extensive schooling and the growing availability of Spanish-language entertainment are the factors most often cited as providing the impetus for wider use of Spanish in Pichátaro. In about 60% of all households, Spanish is reported as the more commonly used language, with only about one-fourth of the households claiming more frequent use of Tarascan. The remainder (16%) report approximately equal use of the two languages. A common pattern is for Tarascan to be spoken among the adults, and Spanish to the children and among the children themselves. One still routinely hears Tarascan in everyday conversations, particularly among women. Tarascan speech continues to be one of the most salient characteristics distinguishing Pichátaro as an Indian community, but it is clear that its use is rapidly declining with each succeeding generation. While three-fourths of all adults are Tarascan speakers, few persons below the age of twenty or twenty-five claim a fluency in the language, although many say that they understand it. Their children, in turn, are unlikely to learn it at all.

The people of Pichátaro have generally had limited opportunity to obtain formal schooling. Only 15% of the adult population has completed the six years of primary school, and only about one in twenty has completed secondary school (three additional years) or more. About one-fourth of the men, and nearly half of the women, have had no schooling at all. At all levels the educational attainment of men is greater than that of women. A little over half of all Pichátaro adults are literate to some degree; this figure includes, as one might expect, a good many more men than women. Before the 1950's the instruction available in Pichátaro covered just the first three years of primary school. The only way in which additional schooling could be obtained was to leave town and attend a government boarding school in Paracho. These days, however, Pichátaro has two six-year primary schools and the beginnings of a secondary school. The proportion of children now attending and completing school is greater than in the past, and the overall level of education is rising.

MAKING A LIVING

Although Pichátaro is primarily an agricultural community, the ways in which its residents make a living are actually fairly diverse. In talking about livelihoods, distinction is often made between "destinies"—one's fixed, regular, and most important work—and "little jobs"—secondary or occasional productive activities. All men have a destiny; most men's livelihoods derive from pursuit of their destiny and one or more little jobs—for example, farmer and resin collector, farmer and board cutter. Table 2.1 gives the proportions of Pichátaro males over fifteen years following each of the most frequently encountered destinies.

Almost three-fourths of all men are farmers—either tillers of their own lands *(agricultores),* sharecroppers *(medieros),* or landless wage laborers in others' fields *(jornaleros).* Agriculture in Pichátaro is almost entirely nonmechanized and therefore dependent upon human and animal energy. No one at the time of our study owned, or had ever owned, a tractor, although a few wealthier families sometimes hired tractor owners from other towns to perform some of the heavier tasks in their fields. Maize is the basic staple of the Pichátaro diet, and by far the most important and frequent crop grown. Smaller amounts of wheat, oats, and barley are sown by some men each year, mainly for sale outside of town or for animal feed.

The remaining destinies are primarily service or manufacturing occupations, most of which are dependent upon the patronage of the farming households. Woodworkers are engaged either in carpentry or as artisans—makers of carved plaques, frames, and figures for sale to tourist shops in Pátzcuaro and Quiroga. Musicians find most of their work in town ceremonial events, such as saints' fiestas, weddings, some funerals, and baptisms, all of which require anywhere from a small group of musicians to a complete band.

Table 2.1. **Male Occupations**

Principal occupation ("destiny")	Number	Percentage
Farmer	554	72.2
Woodworker	33	4.3
Musician	22	2.9
Mason	21	2.7
Merchant	20	2.6
Teacher	16	2.1
Weaver	10	1.3
Butcher	5	0.7
(Other occupations)	86	11.2
Total	767	100.0

Most of the merchants are keepers of small local stores, although a few are truck owners and work at hauling various goods to and from town.

A wide variety of little jobs are pursued, the most important being resin collecting, which is done by members of over half of the households in town. The process itself involves no more than cutting a gash in the side of a pine and placing a cup at the lower end of it to catch the resin as it oozes from the wound. Those who have a stand of trees in Pichátaro's forest lands and exploit them for this purpose make a visit every week or two, depending upon the season, to gather the resin and deliver it to a collection yard where it is bought on a per kilo basis and stored in barrels until being trucked from town.[5]

Another important little job, called "adventuring," is temporary wage labor migration, primarily to the Mexico City area but also to the United States. A number of people report that their first real experience with modern medical treatment occurred while living temporarily at these locations. In a sample of sixty-one household heads questioned on their experiences, about half (thirty-one) had left the area at some time to seek temporary wage labor. On the average they had done so between two and three times, for periods of roughly two months per trip. These trips are usually undertaken when some unusual expense, such as a serious illness or a wedding, makes it necessary to raise a relatively large amount of cash quickly. They usually last only as long as it takes to earn the necessary amount. Such trips, as the adventuring label may suggest, are undertaken with a fair degree of ambivalence; their outcomes are not always certain, and Pichatareños on the whole consider large urban areas such as Mexico City stressful and unsafe places to live. There is a fairly large community of former Pichátaro residents in one area of the capital, and it is through the network of friends and relatives living there that temporary work is found, usually in construction. Temporary labor migration is closely tied to the farming cycle, and most often occurs in the months following planting and weeding, but preceding the harvest in December. In addition to Mexico City migration, about one out of four male heads of households has worked in the United States. Most went during World War II or later, during the time of the bracero program, usually staying for less than a year. In recent times a much smaller number has migrated successfully, apparently due to the greater difficulty and expense involved in illegal entry, as well as the absence of any network of relatives or townspeople in the border area. Interest in work opportunities in the United States, however, remains keen.

Women's occupations are less varied. For 95% of Pichátaro females over fifteen years, the domestic chores of meal preparation, laundering, and child care are the primary occupations. About half of this number take on additional activities such as embroidering, bread making, or weaving to supplement the family's income. Another thirty women are secondarily engaged in commerce, either as streetside vegetable sellers or in working alongside their husbands in operating a store. The other 5% represents twenty-five young women attending post-primary school, eight teachers, and seven women primarily involved in other occupations, including curing and midwifery.

Pichátaro seems materially better off than many rural indigenous Mesoamerican communities. The town has relatively abundant and fertile agricultural lands. There are still small pieces of land in Pichátaro's territory that, although arable, have not been put to use simply because more conveniently located land has always been available. Obviously with increasing population this will change, but it remains true that up until the present Pichátaro has generally had sufficient land to provide for the basic subsistence needs of its population.[6]

Nevertheless, by Mexican national standards, and of course much more so by North American standards, Pichátaro is a poor community. For example, daily wages paid for agricultural work in 1976 were around thirty-five to forty pesos (equivalent to about $3.00 at the then current exchange rate, but about $1.75 after the devaluation of the peso late in 1976). Homes have some amenities: 90% have a piped water source, usually a spigot sprouting up somewhere within the household compound; 60% have electric power; about 50% include a radio among the household possessions; and surprisingly, about one out of seven has a television. On the other hand, of over five hundred of these homes, no more than a handful have indoor plumbing, even fewer have refrigeration equipment, and there is no heating (save for a smoky fire in the kitchen shed), even in the below-freezing nighttime temperatures of December and January. Rats and mice are common pests, and domestic animals, such as chickens and pigs, are kept in household compounds in close association with humans. The community as a whole lacks the resources to provide services such as a sewage system, waste collection and disposal, or public bathing facilities as are found in some larger towns and cities.

At the same time, there is considerable variation in the wealth, and hence the standard of living, of different households. For example, Household A is composed of an older couple, living with a grandson, his wife, and their small son. Their lot has but two structures, both of them tiny shake-walled shacks, barely tall enough for them to stand in. The kitchen includes a three-stone hearth in the center of the dirt floor, one small chair, some clay cooking ware, and a few dishes. The other building has one table (which holds the family saint's image), two vegetable crates that serve as chairs, and some clothing hung on a rope strung across one wall. There is neither water nor electricity. In the rainy season the compound is awash with mud, and the buildings offer only minimal protection from the driving rains, and practically none at all from the bone-chilling nighttime cold. In comparison, consider Household B, also with five members. This is the family of a man who spent several years working as a migrant laborer in the United States. His house is located on the main street of town, and includes a large masonry building that houses his store in front, and within, a fine old *troje* and a handsome, brightly painted masonry house having several rooms. The patio area in front of the house is surfaced with concrete, and has several benches arranged around the edges. Many flowering plants potted in discarded chile cans decorate the area. The house itself has several glassed windows, heavy carved wooden doors, and concrete floors.

Wealth differences such as these are readily acknowledged by informants, who can easily and consistently rank their fellow townsmen in terms of their relative wealth.[7] Such ranking was in fact done.[8] The single feature that most consistently accounts for a given household's position is land ownership. The households that ranked poorest, such as Household A, were all landless. The middle 60–70% of the households are generally land owners, with increasingly greater holdings as one moves to the higher ranks. Those above the median frequently own cattle or sheep, or work at some second occupation in addition to farming. The very wealthiest in the sample, such as Household B, were storekeepers or owners of the better-equipped woodworking shops.

Most households, except perhaps the very wealthiest and those of the storekeepers, do not have large amounts of cash on hand. Surplus cash is often used to buy animals, especially pigs, with the intent of keeping them on hand for quick sale should an emergency arise, such as a serious illness, in which the money were needed. One man, in fact, jokingly referred to a sow he had just bought as his *cuenta de ahorros* ('savings account')! There are no organized credit facilities in Pichátaro or elsewhere used by residents, who must depend upon relatives and ritual kinsmen for loans when a need arises and there is no other way to raise the money. As a last resort, there are a few moneylenders in town who require land,[9] horses, or other property as security, and charge high interest (20–25% per month). Understandably, people are quite reluctant to go to them, and usually do so only in extreme emergencies.

FAMILY LIFE AND PUBLIC LIFE

The most important social group in Pichátaro is the household. It is the basic unit of production and consumption, and is formally recognized as a corporate unit for several purposes. The physical boundaries of the domestic unit are usually quite clear; it typically consists of a number of separate buildings gathered closely together on a fenced lot *(solar),* and has a single hearth regardless of the number of co-resident nuclear (husband-wife) units. Figures from our census show 509 households in Pichátaro, having on the average between five and six members. The composition of these households is varied. The core of most is the nuclear family; 46% of all households are composed solely of a married couple with only unmarried children living with them. Typically additions first occur when the oldest son marries and his wife comes to live in the household, until such time as the new couple is able to acquire a house and establish an independent residence. This cycle of marriage, temporary patrilocality, and subsequent establishment of a new household continues with each successive son until reaching the youngest child, either male or female. After marriage, this couple is expected to remain permanently with the aging parents, upon whose death they will inherit the house and lot. In fact, the composition of about three-fourths of all Pichátaro households is consistent with this developmental pattern. The remaining households represent widows or, much less commonly, widowers, living alone; households basically conforming to the above pattern but with the absence by death of some key member; joint households composed of two married brothers and their respective families; or households composed of highly variable agglomerations of relatives, usually around a nuclear family core, that have resulted from a variety of special circumstances.

Households in Pichátaro are largely self-sufficient economic units.[10] Daily chores are assigned to all members considered old enough to carry them out, with daughters in particular taking up regular household duties much earlier than sons. The main obligations of kin outside of the domestic unit are restricted to participation in special household events such as weddings, funerals, and religious *cargo* fiestas, which I discuss later in this chapter. Close kin are also commonly recruited for help during the harvest; this help is reciprocated. Cooperation between brothers in other agricultural tasks, such as plowing, is fairly common, although there is not the same sort of formal expectation as with the harvest.

Beyond the nuclear family and the domestic unit, the significance of consanguineal and affinal ties quickly gives way to the pseudokinship of the *compadrazgo* system. The essential features of this system of ritual co-parenthood have been described in several works (see Mintz and Wolf 1950; Ravicz 1967). Briefly, for a number of important events in the life of one's child, beginning with baptism, parents choose a married couple (rarely, an individual) to serve as the child's ritual sponsors or godparents. Obviously a godparent-godchild relationship is thus established, but of much greater importance is the relationship that is created between the child's parents and godparents. They are now *compadres* (*compadre* with a man, and *comadre* with a woman), literally co-parents, a relationship of reciprocal aid, trust, and respect. The principal *compadre* ties, such as those of baptism, approach in significance even the closest blood relationship. Ideally, *compadrazgo* ties are established with persons with whom one already has considerable *confianza* ('trust'), and they act merely to cement and formalize that relationship. Perhaps equally often in practice, potential *compadres* are chosen with a more purposeful intent—that of building up a set of allies, bound to each by obligations and expectations of mutual assistance and support. It is largely to his *compadres,* even more than to his closest relatives, that a man may turn for political support, for assistance in carrying out a fiesta obligation, for loans in emergencies, and in other times of need. Thus, an important consideration in the choice of *compadres* is the extent to which a potential contractant is in a position to render such assistance. The more powerful and wealthy men in Pichátaro are naturally quite popular choices and tend to have extensive networks of *compadres* in all parts of town. *Compadre* ties may be created on several occasions in the life of one's child, such as baptism, confirmation, first communion, *la corona* ('the crown'),[11] and marriage. These ties are ranked in importance, and therefore in the strength of the obligations and expectations they entail. Those of baptism are the most significant, followed by those of confirmation and marriage. First communion and *la corona compadres* have proportionately weaker obligations, and relationships between them tend to be less formal than with the preceding types.

Not all *compadre* choices are made solely with the idea of forming a potentially useful alliance. Certainly a great many are made simply out of genuine friendship and esteem, or because parents feel that a particularly well respected or successful person would make a good example for their child. Nevertheless, social relation-

ships in Pichátaro tend strongly to be individualistic and instrumental in nature, as is especially apparent in the institution of the
compadrazgo.

After the household, the next regularly constituted and territo-
rially defined social unit in Pichátaro is the *barrio* ('neighborhood'
or 'ward'). Although historically *barrios* in some Mesoamerican
communities were formed from existing indigenous divisions, it
seems most likely that Pichátaro's seven contiguous *barrios* represent the concentration of a like number of smaller settlements that
occurred during the colonial period. The *barrios* are each named
after a patron saint, and formerly, it is said, each had its own small
chapel and celebrated its saint's day. Currently, however, only San
Miguel *barrio,* the largest, has a chapel and annual fiesta.[12] *Barrio*
membership is on the basis of residence, although members of one
barrio who move as adults to a house located in another often continue to claim membership in the original *barrio;* the children
would subsequently claim membership in the second *barrio.* There
is no strong tendency or preference for *barrio* endogamy, other
than what would normally occur on the basis of propinquity. Neither is there any significant occupational specialization among the
barrios. Each is headed by an elected chief and his assistant, who
are responsible for the coordination of *barrio* activities. These activities include communal labor projects *(faena),* such as repairing
roads, moving houses, cleaning the churchyard, repairing municipal
buildings, and other public works tasks. Participation in communal
labor sometimes becomes the basis for inter-*barrio* rivalry, the
members of one *barrio* claiming that they participate more enthusiastically and frequently than those of another. The annual Sixth
of August fiesta, the largest of the year, is financed on a *barrio,*
rather than an individual sponsor, basis. For a given year, each *barrio* is responsible for providing one part of the fiesta—such as a
band, a *castillo* (fireworks display), decoration for the church—the
particular responsibility rotating from one year to the next.

A more informal but perhaps more significant division exists between the "upper" *(arriba)* and "lower" *(abajo)* halves of town.
This distinction is used more commonly than *barrio* names in referring to locations and directions and reflects what is in many ways a

functional two-*barrio* system in Pichátaro.[13] This division does have some small basis in the geography of the town; the upper part is slightly, and very gradually, higher in elevation. But by no means is it a mere reflection of the local topography. Rather, it represents a real community cleavage, with residents on each side considering themselves as somehow different from those on the other, and along which factionalist politics frequently develop.[14] People living in the lower part of town say that those living "up there" are hard-headed and resistant to new ideas, that they don't speak Spanish well ("if they can't get it across in words, they do it with their fists"), and that, all in all, they are just "different people," even though "we are all of the same pueblo." On the other hand, those living in the upper part of town say that, in comparison with those "below," they are more spirited, more cooperative, and always willing to help each other. To the outsider, there are further apparent differences. Tarascan seems somewhat more widely spoken, and men's clothing styles more traditional (blankets instead of jackets) in the upper part of town. There is a certain degree of antagonism evident between people from the two parts, and it is said that in the past youthful fighting between them was frequent; even entering the opposite part of town was sometimes risky business.

Pichátaro's official governmental structure is dualistic, with separate sets of officials for each of the town's two formal statuses: as a *tenencia* (subordinate town) of the *municipio* of Tingambato, and as a *comunidad indígena* ('indigenous community').[15]

The major administrative units of the state of Michoacán are *municipios,* similar to counties in the United States. *Municipios* are composed of a head town *(cabecera)* and usually several subordinate towns or villages. Pichátaro is such a subordinate town and consequently does not have the full complement of officials *(ayuntamiento)* otherwise associated with towns of its size.[16] In everyday affairs, however, Pichátaro is largely autonomous from the municipal government in Tingambato. Its governing body includes a *jefe de tenencia,* a substitute *jefe,* a secretary, a judge, a commander of the police, and three or four policemen. A principal job of the *jefe* is to mediate between the town and outside governmental agencies and officials. His duties include handling official town correspondence, usually in the form of petitions to the federal government, as well as coordinating communal work projects, providing support for the schools, and organizing the major town fiestas. The substitute *jefe* has few duties, except in the event that the *jefe* becomes unable or unwilling to continue in office. The secretary is the only paid official, and as the job requires writing and typing skills, he tends to serve for several years. Since *jefes* rotate through town government on a yearly basis, and usually have no previous experience in these affairs, it is the secretary who provides the experience and continuity and who does a good deal of the actual work. The office of judge is a fairly minor one, which apparently had not been filled during 1977. The police occasionally patrol the town on weekends and during fiestas when drunks are likely to cause trouble.

The office of *jefe* is unpaid and requires a substantial time investment, as he is expected to be around the *jefatura* (town hall) a good part of the day. Since the position carries responsibilities but little actual power, and since the *jefe* usually receives a good deal of criticism regardless of how the job is carried out, men are not anxious to run for the office and usually must be cajoled into accepting it. Candidates for *jefe* are nominated with no party affiliation and voted on at a general town meeting presided over by the *presidente municipal* from Tingambato (in one of his few yearly visits to Pichátaro). The runner-up in the voting becomes the substitute *jefe*, and the remaining officials are appointed by the new *jefe*.

Pichátaro's second legal identity is as an "indigenous community," an administrative status introduced in the colonial period and still recognized by the state government (Moone 1969:61; Carrasco 1952). The designation refers primarily to the form of land tenure; lands in Pichátaro are, from the state's point of view, communally held rather than *ejido* (a government land grant made as part of Mexico's post-Revolutionary land reform program) or privately owned. The main official of the *comunidad indígena* is the *representante del pueblo*,[17] who has as his primary duty the administration of the town's lands. The *representante* ordinarily serves for a three-year term and is assisted by a secretary and other minor officials. He assigns particular areas of the communal forest lands to individuals for resin collecting and takes charge of the annual collection of a small contribution each household pays for rights to use the forests, and toward meeting the tax the town as a whole must pay to the state as rent on its agricultural lands.

There is neither a set hierarchy of civil offices through which individuals pass in reaching the position of *representante* or *jefe* nor any necessity that town officials should be selected from among those who have also served in religious posts. The system of office holding in Pichátaro lacks the ladder structure described in some Indian communities in other areas of Mesoamerica, especially Chiapas and highland Guatemala.

Politics in Pichátaro persistently tend toward factionalism, frequently coalescing along the upper-lower division of the town, and are characterized by a continuing search for one single representative, one upon whom everyone will agree, and who will unite all segments of the town and lead it forward to greater prosperity. Needless to say, such a person has yet to appear. Routinely town officials are criticized for doing nothing and are often suspected of corruption. Consensus on communitywide issues is infrequent, since the community structure makes effective leadership difficult. For example, in 1975 the state government offered to help construct a small health center in Pichátaro, but two years later the work had still not begun; no agreement could be reached on where the center should be located, and there were conflicting claims over rights to the location most often proposed.

MAKING FIESTA

Pichatareños devote their time not only to making a living but also to "making fiesta." Two major kinds of fiestas take place in Pichátaro: community fiestas, ostensibly to celebrate particular Catholic religious holidays, in which people say they participate as a means of "enjoying life"; and those fiestas marking important events in the life cycles of individuals—especially baptisms and weddings—in which people participate in order to "accompany relatives."

Making fiesta is a central activity in Pichátaro. The number of days devoted specifically to just the major, communitywide fiestas occurring during the year amounts to slightly more than a month's time. Add to this the days devoted to preparations for these occasions, and the estimate is closer to a month and a half. Finally, including all of the weddings, baptisms, house-roofings, and other minor fiestas inevitably attended during the year, the total is at least two months out of every year spent largely in preparing for and attending fiestas. While other activities are of course not completely suspended on all of these days, these figures, along with the obvious enthusiasm of residents as they discuss upcoming fiestas, emphasize the significance of these events in Pichátaro life.

The annual cycle of communitywide fiestas includes no fewer than a dozen, the most important being the three-week long period in which Christmas is celebrated; the fiesta of Corpus in June; and the Sixth of August fiesta, Pichátaro's largest, in honor of a small, highly venerated image in the town church, the "Precious Blood of Christ." Pichátaro's formal ceremonial organization consists of a set of yearly offices *(cargos),* almost all associated with a particular fiesta.[18] The most important and costly of these is the office of *colector,* which carries responsibility for ceremonial activities at Christmas and for the care and display of the image of the child Jesus throughout the year. The *colector* is named by the town priest, and is either someone who has requested the office or, if no one has volunteered, someone chosen by the priest. Because of the expense involved usually only wealthier residents are selected to serve in this office. *Colectores* are most often men (a woman held the office in 1972) and tend to have previously held no other religious offices. The *colector* is assisted by a senior and a junior *regidor,* who also serve for one year. Following the *colector* and *regidores* in importance is the *mayordomo,* whose main duty is the maintenance of an ever-burning oil lamp in the church. This office is usually requested. Of similar importance is the position of the *hainde,* who has the responsibility of providing the large quantity of palm necessary for the Palm Sunday procession.

Each of these religious offices, while not a part of the official church structure, are nonetheless under direct control of the town priest. But there is a second class of religious offices in Pichátaro existing entirely apart from the church organization, the '*cargos* of the outside fiestas'. Of the principal occupational (not all are full-time destinies) groups in Pichátaro each has its own patron saint—the farmers' is San Isidro, the carpenters' is San José, the honey collectors' is San Anselmo, the musicians' is Santa Cecilia, and so on. Each of these groups names a *carguero* to serve for a year. His duties include the care of the saint's image, and, on the appropriate date, the sponsorship of a fiesta in honor of the saint. This is attended by all of the members of the group, and usually many others. The two largest outside fiestas of this type are those of San Isidro and Santa Cecilia. The San Isidro fiesta is in many ways a smaller version of the Corpus fiesta, and since most Pichátaro men are farmers, it approaches communitywide proportions. The fiesta of Santa Cecilia is also large, because, it is said, "musicians like to make fiesta." Of these yearly offices, that of San Isidro is generally ranked as the most important—apparently because it is the most costly. Individuals do not progress through these offices; they are usually affiliated with but a single group.

CHANGES IN PICHATARO

In the past, residents often say, Pichátaro was a "forgotten town," largely ignored by and receiving little assistance from the government. This image has begun to change somewhat in recent years, however, as Pichátaro has witnessed a number of efforts to promote changes. In fact, between 1975 and 1977, no fewer than six government development agencies were active, to varying degrees, in the town.

Investments facilitating communication with the wider society have brought about some of the more significant recent changes. Most important among these was the construction in 1971–1972 of a dirt road connecting the town with the Pátzcuaro-Uruapan highway. With it came direct bus service to Pátzcuaro, from which it is relatively easy to travel to other cities in the region and beyond. Whereas formerly a trip to Pátzcuaro was an all day or overnight affair, a round trip could now be accomplished in a single morning. The most immediate effect was a dramatic drop in attendance at the Erongarícuaro market, as the much larger Friday and Sunday markets in Pátzcuaro became the focus of Pichátaro commerce. Dozens of women have since begun baking bread for sale through this new outlet, and craft production has substantially increased. The new road has also been the single most important factor in increasing the accessibility of Western medical treatment; before this, people say that curing was nearly always accomplished with folk remedies, as it was impossible to transport a seriously ill person from town.

The electrification of the town in the 1950's also brought significant changes. Nighttime activities increased, and first radios, then televisions, became more common. This increased media exposure now gives many residents an awareness of issues seemingly as distant from town life as the supersonic transport controversy and U.S. presidential politics. The frequent media advertising of patent medicines and other cures has undoubtedly had some effect on the present state of medical knowledge in Pichátaro.

The two agencies of the Mexican government most directly involved in change programs in Pichátaro at the time of the study were the Cultural Missions Department and the National Indian Institute.

Cultural Missions, a program of the federal Ministry of Public Education, are essentially community development teams. They attempt to improve the local standard of living, thus facilitating the national integration of heretofore marginal rural communities (see Ewald 1967:496–501). The Pichátaro Mission, which established itself in town in August 1975, consisted of eight teachers specialized in nursing, agriculture, recreation, music, social work, carpentry, masonry, and crafts. A chief was responsible for the direction of the group's activities. Attached to the group was another teacher in charge of a public reading room. The Pichátaro Mission's methods included formal classes, practical demonstrations, home visits, and organization of various community projects. In spite of its efforts, however, at the end of the first year the Mission had met with minimal success. Residents generally believed that little had been accomplished. Classes were poorly attended, and several planned projects had not been carried out. Less than one-fourth of a sample of fifty households surveyed reported any significant involvement in the Mission's activities.

Several factors appear to have contributed to the failure of the Mission to achieve widespread community interest and participation. Residents were often put off by teachers' occasionally haughty manner and poor preparation in their specialties; as one man said, "They went around a lot making the appearance of being maestros, but they didn't do anything!" The Mission was also plagued by organizational problems: the original chief resigned after a few months amid much gossip; it was several weeks before his replacement arrived, and even longer before routine work was again begun. But perhaps the most fundamental error accounting for this particular Mission's lack of success was its failure to develop a significant personal relationship with town residents. As was discussed earlier, social relationships in Pichátaro tend strongly to be individualistic, and people seek assistance largely on a one-to-one basis, from persons with whom they have an established tradition of mutual cooperation and trust. The teachers of the Mission, on the other hand, tended to stay close together, to spend most of their free time with each other, and attempted to deal with the residents primarily on a collective, and often classroom, basis.

The second government agency with programs involving Pichátaro is the National Indian Institute (I.N.I.). The town is included in the zone of influence of the new Lake Region Coordinating Center in Pátzcuaro. Until 1975 the town was included, but apparently only marginally, in the zone of the older Cherán Coordinating Center, which seems to have been involved in few activities in Pichátaro. The Pátzcuaro Center, however, was showing signs of greater interest, perhaps partially because its director was born in Pichátaro and still maintains a house in town. As of 1977, the main I.N.I. activity had been the operation of a small medical post, staffed by a single nurse. Shortly before our departure in August of that year, the Pátzcuaro Center had also arranged for an advanced medical student from the University of Michoacán in Morelia to spend weekends holding consultations in town. (These programs

are discussed in greater detail in Chapter Five.) In other areas, the
I.N.I. Center, along with a state artisan development program, has
been active in organizing several events during the Sixth of August
fiesta designed to attract more outsiders and tourists and promote
the town's craft industry.

A variety of other governmental agencies have sporadically initiated more limited projects in Pichátaro. Between 1975 and 1977
these included a model apiary, demonstration plots showing results
of new maize fertilization recommendations, and an as yet unsuccessful project promoting potato production.

THE WIDER CONTEXT

Ethnically, nearly all of Pichátaro's three thousand residents are
considered by the larger society, and by and large consider themselves, as Indian, and the Tarascan language remains commonly
spoken in the town. Economically, the majority of Pichatareños depend upon subsistence maize agriculture. Politically, the town is
near the low end of the Mexican governmental hierarchy, and because of its subordinate municipal status it lacks wider influence;
internally, there is a tendency toward factionalism, and effective
community leadership is often difficult to achieve. Spiritually, the
people are participants in a generalized folk Catholicism, and town
life is largely measured through a rich and extensive annual fiesta
cycle.

Pichátaro is, by most standards, a poor community, and this is
generally true of the Tarascan area as a whole. Certainly its poverty is a powerful factor in determining the overall health of its
residents. Moreover, the economically disadvantageous position of
most townspeople strongly affects decisions on how to treat illness.
In a real way, then, an understanding of health care and medical
choice in Pichátaro requires some consideration of the factors involved in the perpetuation of relative poverty. For this, we must
look beyond Pichátaro's boundaries, to its relationship with the
larger Mexican society that surrounds it, and consider an additional identity that the town shares with the rural indigenous sector in general—that of marginality.

Marginality implies an absence of effective participation in the national economy and society. Since rural poverty is generally viewed as a direct consequence of marginality, the explanation of poverty must be phrased in terms of those factors constraining a community's (or region's) national participation. Two different explanations are evident in the literature. The first relates marginality to factors internal to the community. Some reputed characteristics of marginal people, such as peasant conservatism and resistance to change, or of their cultures, such as fatalistic world views and tradition-bound social structures, are seen as impediments to change and as barriers to a people's taking advantage of development opportunities available to them. In this view, more effective integration and the consequent reduction of poverty can be achieved by educative programs—such as those of the Cultural Missions—which aim to re-tool the people's productive skills and reorient their outlook and cultural identity to that of the national society.

A second view, however, holds that marginality results from a community's peripheral position in relation to the concentration of wealth and economic decision making in the society; it is excluded from effective control over the system and from participation in its benefits (Adams 1974:45). This exclusion from full participation in the national economy results in poverty. Such peoples are integrated into the national economy in the sense that they are dependent upon cash for part of their livelihood (Whitten and Szwed 1970:43), and insofar as they provide a necessary reserve labor supply for national development (as do, for example, the Pichatareños who undertake temporary wage labor migration to the Mexico City area). But because they are structurally far removed from the centers of power over economic resources, they do not share in the economic benefits of development. Barkin (1975), for example, has documented how economic development in the hot country of Michoacán has had the effect of transferring control over resources from the local community to the wealthier urban sector of the nation possessing the capital necessary for participation in the new system of production. Thus, in this view, marginality and the poverty accompanying it are a consequence of national development;

characteristics of marginal communities such as "resistance to change" and general "backwardness," rather than serving as impediments to national participation and integration, are in fact effects of the institutionalized denial of genuine opportunities for such participation. Such institutionalized exclusion is part of a pattern of Mexico's national development in recent decades; it has also been a constant feature of the history of rural-urban and indigenous-Hispanic relations since the Conquest, as Margolies has so eloquently demonstrated in the case of a village in Mexico state (Margolies 1975).

To review the history of Pichátaro's relationship with the wider society, and to document the specific conditions responsible for the town's current economic position, would be beyond the scope of the present study. We have raised these issues here because the contrast between explanations of marginality that point to internal "cultural peculiarities" of peasant communities, and those that cite features of inequality and exclusion in the relations of such communities with the larger society, is analogous to a current debate concerning the reactions of rural people to modern medicine. Is the low utilization of modern medicine by rural Third World peoples primarily due to the influence of so-called cultural factors, such as traditional beliefs and values, or is it due to factors of inaccessibility and exclusion? By the last chapter of this book, we shall be in a good position to examine these issues critically.

3

Medical Beliefs in
Pichátaro

To understand the rationale underlying illness treatment decisions in Pichátaro also requires examination of the medical beliefs characteristic of the community in which they occur. This
study is, therefore, an analysis of the Pichátaro medical system as a
whole. The concept of a medical system as the focus of ethnomedi-
cal inquiry is now a general one, and although definitions vary (see,
for example, Dunn 1976; Fabrega 1972; Foster and Anderson 1978;
Leslie 1976), it is usually conceived of as: 1. a culturally relative
system of knowledge that forms the basis for actions relating to illness; and 2. the institutional arrangements within which these actions occur. This and the following chapter are concerned with the
first of these two categories—that body of knowledge used in explaining the occurrence of illness and in evaluating its potential
consequences.

Details are largely unavailable concerning the historical development of present-day medical beliefs in Pichátaro. Several works
(see Foster 1953; Logan 1973) have described the introduction of
sixteenth-century Spanish medicine, and especially the humoral
theory of illness, into post-Conquest Mesoamerica, and this process
seems to have been more than ordinarily complete in the case of the
Tarascan region. As in many areas of modern Tarascan culture (see
R. Beals 1946:210–211), few if any clearly identifiable pre-Conquest
beliefs and practices concerning illness are to be found. At the same
time, it should not be assumed that ideas about illness causation
and process in Pichátaro have remained unchanged since their
introduction, free from local development and differentiation.
Rather, the particular context into which they were introduced and
their subsequent reworking have resulted in a contemporary sys-

tem of illness beliefs that, while having many basic similarities with those reported from elsewhere in Mesoamerica, also incorporates a number of distinctive features.

THE BODILY BASIS OF ILLNESS

In order to understand Pichatareño illness beliefs it is necessary to consider their view of the human body and how it works. Folk knowledge of bodily structure and functioning, and conceptions of how different agents and forces may impinge on this functioning and create illness, form an important class of information from which individuals draw in evaluating symptoms, assessing their seriousness, and ultimately deciding upon a course of action to be followed in providing treatment.

Data on Mesoamerican body concepts are rather few, although— assuming Pichátaro is representative in this regard—many illness beliefs are not comprehensible without inquiry into their ethnoana- tomical and ethnophysiological basis. There are several analyses of body part classifications (see Brown et al. 1976 and Friedrich 1969; see also Brown 1976 for additional references), but these deal with external parts, such as legs, arms, and hands almost exclusively, while it is the internal parts that are most significant for illness be- liefs. The main exceptions are the studies of Adams (1952), Holland (1963), and Douglas (1969), all dealing with communities in the Mayan area. Douglas's work is of special interest, as comparison of his findings with those reported in this study reveals several significant similarities, particularly in regard to the digestive proc- ess. It seems, then, that parts of the present description may have some generality beyond the specific case of Pichátaro (see also Adams and Rubel 1967:334).

Two techniques were used in gathering the data reported in this section. First, eight people were asked to name "all of the parts that we have inside of us," a procedure that usually resulted in a listing of ten to fifteen terms. A simple drawing showing an outline of the human body was then brought out, and the informant was asked to sketch in the general shape, size, and location of all the parts she or he had named. After initial coaxing (considerable in some cases), all informants agreed to attempt the task. A general discussion of each part's functioning followed the sketching. It was not possible to question all eight informants on exactly the same points; some had not mentioned particular parts, and some relevant queries had not been discovered until late in the interview series. Therefore, we compiled a twenty-eight-item open-ended interview schedule—designed to cover the major details in the initial interviews—and made a return visit with each informant. To the extent that these eight individuals represent the community in general, it becomes possible to indicate the degree of consensus or disagreement existing on several issues.

Sources of knowledge about the body are several but indirect, since no one reported having actually seen the interior of the human body. Because of this lack of direct evidence, beliefs about its structure are frequently imprecise. Perhaps the most important kind of information comes from rough analogies with animals. Cows butchered in the street in front of meat shops provide a view of their internal structure. Pigs, regarded as being the most like humans in their anatomy, are raised in many households and subsequently butchered. Among other sources, people commonly have in their homes popular "medical" guides (often scientifically inaccurate) and school textbooks which include anatomical diagrams. One woman mentioned a large anatomical chart she had viewed at the stall of a medicine vendor in the Pátzcuaro market. Visiting medicine sellers (see Chapter Five) often give elaborate anatomical explanations of the maladies they profess to cure with their remedies. Many concepts informants report are undoubtedly based on no more than everyday bodily sensations, such as the cooling effect of evaporating sweat, the feeling of fullness in the area of the stomach after a meal, or the bleeding and pain that occur when one is injured.

We will now construct a generalized Pichátaro view of the human body, incorporating somewhat more detail than any one informant provided, but with which all informants would more or less agree. First, we will examine the concept of *fuerza* and the notion of balance, both of which are ubiquitous in folk explanations of bodily structure, function, and pathology. Then we will briefly describe each of the major internal parts. Some parts are known only vaguely, whereas others are of special interest. Generally, the greatest detail exists concerning those parts that are directly involved in essential body processes. We will discuss several of these processes, including digestion, circulation, temperature regulation, and sleep.

Fuerza ('strength' or 'vigor'), is the basis of bodily functioning. Most body parts and processes may be understood in terms of their role in its provision, distribution, or utilization. *Fuerza* is obtained from the food and air taken into the body, and dissipated through activity and, at times, illness. To be active, to accomplish one's work, requires that the body have available to it this necessary "fuel." *Fuerza* is also an innate quality, and different individuals have characteristically different stores of it. Men are thought to have more *fuerza* than women, adults more than children. In the aging process one gradually loses the *fuerza* to resist illness, until one dies.

The body also requires that a balance between several opposing forces or tendencies be maintained for its normal functioning—such as the balance between "hotness" and "coldness." In a healthy body these two qualities are equally present. An excess of either, which can be brought about in a number of ways, may lead to illness. The necessity of equilibrium maintenance, however, is not confined to the "hot-cold" qualities, but applies in several other areas as well: one must eat enough food but not too much, as this can "do you damage"; one's stomach needs a certain number of worms, but too many are harmful; one should try not to feel sad, as this can lead to illness, but too much happiness can also make one sick; and one should have desires, but not too strong since, if unfulfilled, one may fall ill.

It is evident in these examples that there is generally no distinction made between physical and emotional causes of illness. The two are believed to be intricately interwoven; the attribution of illness to upsetting or otherwise strong emotional experiences is a salient feature of Pichatareño folk medicine.

The Major Internal Parts

In this section, each of the major internal body parts, and any illnesses specifically associated with them, are briefly described. Figures 3.1 and 3.2 give an approximate idea of their size and locations, as conceived of by one representative informant, a forty-two-year-old woman who neither reads nor writes. Notice that what is being described is the local theory of bodily structure and functioning that may or may not be in accord with the Western biomedical view.

The *pulmones* ('lungs') are thought of as a pair of compact, almost musclelike organs located in the area of the shoulders, just below the surface of the back. While over half of the informants implicated the lungs in breathing, by far the most important function attributed to them is in providing strength to the upper torso and arms. Commonly they were described as "providing strength for work" and as "sustaining the body." Due to their supposed location, pains in the area of the chest are usually attributed to the heart rather than the lungs. Any ache or pain in the upper back, however, such as might result from hours of kneading bread dough or chopping wood, is likely to be attributed to the lungs. Infirmity in later years is often thought to result from such hard work which has "finished off" the lungs.

The *corazón* ('heart') is generally considered the most important part in the body, as it is primarily responsible, through its blood circulation function, for the distribution of *fuerza*. One of the most important factors affecting the heart's functioning is one's emotional state. While physical pain (as from a wound) is felt in or "arrives at" the head, emotional "pains" are felt directly in the heart. It is thought that one's troubles, worries, and sorrows may, over time, result in "sickness of the heart." Two other parts, the *bofe* ('lung') and the *hígado* ('liver'), are said to be "along with the heart, to help it work," and no independent function is attributed to them. Several people described how the liver may be damaged from excessive alcohol, which thereby impedes the functioning of the heart as well.

The *hiel* or *bilis* ('gall bladder') is said by some to be closely asso-

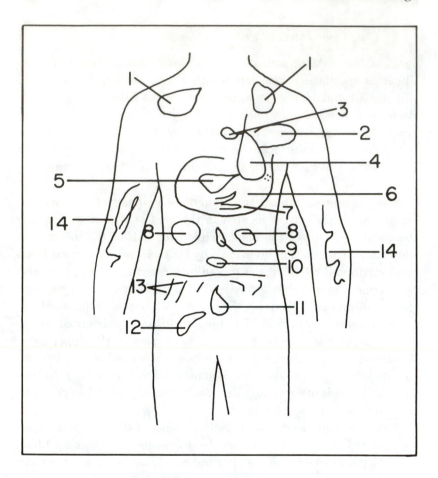

Key

1. *pulmones*—'lungs'
2. *bofe*—'lung'
3. *hiel* or *bilis*—'gall' (bladder)
4. *corazón*—'heart'
5. *hígado*—'liver'
6. *estómago*—'stomach'
7. *tripas*—'guts'
8. *riñones*—'kidneys'
9. *bazo*—'spleen'
10. *latido*—'pulsating ball'
11. *vejiga*—'bladder'
12. *matriz*—'womb' (women only)
13. *nervios*—'nerves'*
14. *venas*—'blood vessels'*
    *Found in all parts of the body

Figure 3.1. **One Informant's View of Human Anatomy**

ciated with the *bofe* and liver and, like them, to further aid the functioning of the heart. Others separate it from these, or even specify both a *hiel* and *bilis* as two distinct parts, the latter being located lower in the abdomen. In any case, no regular function is attributed to the gall bladder. Rather, its significance lies in its potential for causing illness. It is said to contain a liquid, described as "bile" or simply as a "water" which, if the bladder opens up, spreads to all parts of the body causing illness and even death. This release may occur in one of two ways: from strong emotions, such as fright, joy or anger; or from having an intense desire for something which is not realized. Since the "poison" that is released is not localized, the symptoms of the illness they produce (also called *bilis*) are usually nonspecific and diffuse. Accordingly, vague somatic complaints are often diagnosed as *bilis,* and since upsetting experiences are much a part of life in Pichátaro, it is usually not difficult to isolate the cause. Again, we have evidence of the considerable significance Pichatareños place on emotional causes of illness.

The *estómago* ('stomach') and *tripas* ('intestines') work as a unit in receiving food and extracting its *fuerza* for the body's use. Food arrives at the stomach and is then passed to the intestines. There is some disagreement concerning where the actual processing of the food occurs, but most informants specified the intestine. Some people distinguish between the large and small intestine, but there are no specific ideas about their different functions. The role of the intestines in the elimination of wastes is well known. An area of the stomach of particular concern is the point at which the esophagus joins it, the "mouth of the stomach." The stomach in general, and especially this area of it, is considered to be secondary to the heart as a receiver of emotional pains. *Cólico* (sharp stomach pains), vomiting, and diarrhea are all recognized as potential results of strong emotional experiences.

The *riñones* ('kidneys'), located at each side of the waist, are functional analogues of the lungs, as they provide strength to the lower back and legs. Again evident is the idea of a part that provides the general energy and strength required by a particular area of the body. The reasoning here appears to be as follows: the area where the kidneys are believed to be located often aches after heavy lifting or lengthy walking; therefore the kidneys must have provided the *fuerza* for these activities. In general, any low back pain is likely to be attributed to the kidneys. Impaired walking abilities, which sometimes accompany old age, are thought caused by "bad kidneys."

Concepts concerning the *bazo* ('spleen') and the *vejiga* ('bladder') are somewhat ambiguous, but it is clear that they are involved with ingested liquids. Some informants contend that water when drunk first arrives in the *bazo* and then makes its way to the bladder, where it is stored until urination. Others claim that these are simply two names for the same thing. They are of no great importance in illness explanations.

The *latido* ("pulsating ball"; literally 'palpitation') is an interesting body part described as a small ball located behind the navel. Under normal circumstances it has little function. However, if one does not eat enough, or delays a meal too long, the *latido* will "rise up" from its usual position and travel as far as the "mouth of the stomach," to begin jumping or pulsating and perhaps provoke vomiting.[1] This is said also to occur when one eats disagreeable foods. In less extreme cases, when the *latido* rises up only slightly, it is seen as serving to "call the appetite." The *latido* thus presents another case, like the gall bladder, of a part thought to have no major function other than to cause sickness if one is careless. The *latido* responds both to short-term eating delays, as when one is caught in the rain and returns home late from the fields, and longer, chronic undernourishment. Some adults who frequently complain of *latido* attribute their discomfort to the years of hunger they suffered as a child. The symptoms of such an episode of *latido* are generally vague, apart from the pounding or skipping in the lower chest, and may involve withdrawal from normal activities, general uncommunicativeness, and thoughts of *la muerte* ('death').[2]

The *venas* ('blood vessels') are recognized for their function in carrying blood, and are said to exist in all parts of the body. There is no distinction between arteries and veins, but one particular vein, the *vena gruesa* ('big vein'; the aorta?), was distinguished by some. *Nervios* ('nerves') are described as cordlike entities also found in all parts of the body. No distinction is made between nerves, tendons, and ligaments. The most general contrast between *venas* and *nervios* is that the former carry blood (and, some say, air), whereas the latter do not. A few say, however, that both carry blood. The *nervios* function generally as cables which bind the body together and connect muscles to the parts they move. To a lesser extent *venas* also contribute to these functions. Accordingly, aches and strains following heavy work are often described as due to "stretched" nerves and veins.

Apart from the *matríz* ('womb') in women, the two sexes are not thought to differ greatly in internal structure. Some informants felt that the lungs and blood vessels of women are smaller, and that men have characteristically heavier blood. The main contrast, however, is that men are said to possess greater *fuerza,* are more resistant, and are able to do harder work than women.[3] In these ways women are considered (by both male and female informants) "less complete" and "more simple."

There is general agreement that the head contains at least two parts or organs—the *sesos* ('brains'), located at the top of the head, and the *cerebro* ('brain' or 'cerebrum'), located at the base of the neck (see Figure 3.2). Some informants listed a third part, the *sentido* ('senses'), located in the front of the head. Several processes are said to take place in these parts, or else they provide the *fuerza* for the given ability, including thought, memory, hearing, speech, sight, and taste. Further, the different parts are functionally specialized, and although there is little overall agreement on precisely which one is responsible for what, some generalizations are possible. Thought is considered by most to occur in the *cerebro*. There is no specific theory of how this takes place, but blood is said to flow rapidly through this part when one thinks intensely. The *cerebro* is also thought to be involved in speech, since people who receive blows to that area are rendered speechless. Similarly, the memory must be located in the *sesos,* since by tapping on that area of the head when trying to recall something, the memory can be "jarred loose." The *sentido* is said to provide "strength" for the eyes to see, apparently on the basis of its location at the front of the head. Another recognized part of the head is the *mollera* (the 'crown' or 'fontanel'), the area of the skull immediately above the *sesos*. No par-

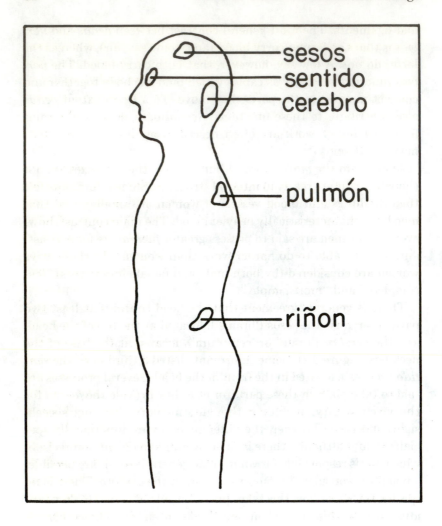

Figure 3.2. **Side View**

ticular function is assigned to it, but it can cause lack of appetite, hearing loss, and loss of vision if it "falls down," an affliction *(mollera caída)* usually confined to children. Apart from their specific functions, the interior parts of the head are also said generally to "fill the head like *masa* ('dough')," "support the veins of vision," and "give strength to the neck."

Some Bodily Processes—Digestion and Nutrition

The parts involved in the Pichátaro view of bodily alimentation are the stomach, intestines, the *bazo,* the bladder, and indirectly the "veins." All contribute to the process whereby the strength contained in food is transferred to the body for use. Let us consider this process, giving special attention to some of the nutritional beliefs that follow from the way in which it is conceptualized.

Some informants believe that there are two tubes passing from the mouth, one of which carries food, the other drink.[4] In this view the two may arrive at separate locations—food in the stomach and water in the *bazo* (or bladder, according to some)—or both may arrive at and mix in the stomach. The remaining informants speak of a single tube through which both pass. In either case, the food mixture then goes to the intestines. At this point, informants consistently explain the digestive process in terms remarkably analogous to the operation of a *molino de nixtamál* ('corn grinding mill'), often describing the intestine as *el molino.* What occurs here is the extraction of the essence of the food, the *mero alimento* ('real' or 'true food'), believed to be a kind of juice in which the strength of the food is concentrated. The juice then passes through the intestines into the veins, which carry it to all parts of the body, providing strength for work and other activity.

An important corollary of this view is that the nutritive value of different foods—the amount of *fuerza* they provide—is considered directly related to their wetness or juiciness. For example, fresh meat, milk, eggs, fresh fish, *čuripu* (boiled meat and cabbage in a chile-seasoned broth), and *sopa de pasta* (noodle soup) are all considered to be highly nutritious and strength-giving foods because they contain a lot of juice. On the other hand, dry *habas* (broadbeans), cheese, dried fish, and meat preserved by drying are considered to have little food value because they largely lack the essential juiciness. The method of preparation may, however, overcome these deficiencies: dried beans can provide considerable *fuerza* when prepared by boiling, which adds moisture. Occasionally some foods are described as containing *mucha vitamina* ('much vitamin'), but this concept is identical to that of *fuerza*.

The equation of juiciness with *fuerza* is true only for items that are classified as *alimentos* ('food').[5] This category is more restricted than the English "food," since most items which are not eaten as part of a meal are not classified as an *alimento*. Thus oranges, although certainly juicy, are not regarded as providing large amounts of *fuerza* because they are not a kind of *alimento*. More specifically, then, it is juicy *alimentos* that provide strength. The juicy-dry distinction[6] is not related to the "hot" and "cold" qualities that foods also have; juicy strength-giving foods may be either "hot," such as pork, or "cold," such as fresh fish.

It is apparent, then, that an emphasis on the juicy qualities of food follows directly from beliefs about how the body utilizes food and extracts its strength-giving properties. Such an equation of juiciness and nutritive value has not been widely reported for the area, perhaps due to the aforementioned scarcity of data on Mesoamerican ethnoanatomical and ethnophysiological concepts. It is significant that one of the few works that does address these issues, Douglas's study from Santiago Atitlán in Guatemala, presents a similar equation, differing only in the details of the various body parts' roles in the process: "The stomach is said to be directly connected to the heart in such a way that the liquid (or strength) of the ingested food is extracted in the stomach and passes directly to the heart and into the blood" (1969:265). It seems that the concept may have some degree of generality beyond the specific case of Pichátaro.

The juicy-dry principle affects the acceptance of new dietary items, a good illustration being the differential adoption of vitamin supplements in Pichátaro. In terms of their effect on and utilization by the body, vitamins are conceptually identical to the juice extracted from foods in the process of digestion. Accordingly, vitamin tonics and injected vitamins are widely regarded as valuable and as particularly useful in building up one's *fuerza* after an illness. Many, in fact, consider such preparations to be a form of concentrated food juice. On the other hand, vitamin tablets, while available, are seldom if ever used because they lack the juiciness considered to be their essence; they are an enigma for reasons that are now apparent.

Occasionally an erroneous equation of juiciness and nutritive value can have severe and unfortunate consequences. Among that minority of Pichátaro women who bottle-feed their infants, powdered infant formulas or powdered milk are sometimes not available due to their cost. What is often considered an acceptable substitute is a mixture of corn meal or even commercially produced corn starch and water. Corn is a prototypical *alimento,* and when prepared in such a moisture-rich form it has all of the attributes of strength-giving food. Of course, the consequences of this practice for the infant's growth and general health are quite serious.

Other important components of nutritional beliefs in Pichátaro are the *solitaria* ('tapeworm') and *lombrices* ('stomach worms'). A person may or may not have a tapeworm, but everyone is said to have stomach worms. The latter are considered essential for their function in "calling the appetite"—calling one's attention to the fact that he should eat. A total lack of worms is thought dangerous because one then loses his appetite and does not eat properly. On the other hand, too many worms can consume too much food and make one thin. They are then a necessary evil; informants explain that they serve to "do damage" and to "offend the stomach," but that nevertheless they are essential for the maintenance of the body's strength. Tapeworms acquire different preferences in different people and thereby lead those having them to overindulge in a certain type of food or drink. One woman explains that her husband has a *solitaria chingadera* (politely, a "drunkard's tapeworm") that continually demands alcohol; the result is that he drinks excessively. Initially tapeworms have no preferences, but slowly they begin to acquire a taste for a certain food that their host eats a lot; they become accustomed to it, and then begin to demand it. *Diabéticos* ('diabetics') are said to be the victims of tapeworms that constantly demand sweets. The origin of tapeworms and stomach worms is unclear. Some say people are born with them ("even from the first day, we are crying for food"); others contend that they are acquired later.

Most residents of Pichátaro believe that if food is to provide strength, it must be eaten at the proper time. In particular, if one waits too long after feelings of hunger begin, the hunger may "pass" and the food will no longer do any good; it is thought that an *aire* ('air') enters the stomach and blocks proper passage of the food. (I have already discussed another possible effect of eating delays—involving the *latido*.)

Circulation and the Blood

The circulation of the blood is viewed as an essential process, as it is the means by which *fuerza* is supplied to all areas of the body. The condition of the parts associated with this function (the heart, blood, veins) is accordingly of great importance for the maintenance of health. The heart is considered to be by far the most important internal bodily part. It is often described as the "pump" or "motor" of the body, and its function in circulating the blood through the veins is well known.

The blood is said to be composed of water and the juice supplied by food, and must be continually augmented with new supplies of juice in order to maintain its strength. Accordingly, loss of blood and poor diet (resulting in "damaged blood") are serious threats to health because they reduce the body's store of *fuerza* and its ability to distribute it. There is some controversy over whether blood, once lost, is replaceable. Some contend that bleeding results in a permanent deficiency and loss of strength. One woman, who has little strength for work, speaks and walks slowly, and is generally weak and phlegmatic, attributes her condition to the heavy bleeding she experienced with the birth of her last child. However, most people questioned on this believe that the supply of blood could be augmented, although slowly, through a diet rich in juicy foods, and with vitamin tonics. In any event, a loss of blood in any quantity is a matter of great concern.

Individuals may vary in the quality of the blood, some having characteristically light or thin blood, others heavy or dark blood. Thin blood is said to "carry" illness more easily, and people having it are thought generally less resistant to illness. In cases of *mal de ojo* ('evil eye') the quality of the infant's blood determines which of the two forms of this illness he will experience.

Temperature Regulation

One of the basic principles of Pichatareño medical beliefs is that of the necessity for a proper balance between hot and cold forces in the body. It is recognized that weather extremes, exertion, inactivity and other factors may act to change this balance and threaten health. Three bodily processes—breathing, sweating, and shivering—are believed to be involved in the correction of such imbalances in the normal individual.

The role of breathing in cooling the body is emphasized in the views of Pichatareños who observe that breathing becomes more rapid during periods of heavy work and other heat-producing activities. Opinion is divided on where the inspired cooling air arrives; some say the lungs, others the stomach. In either case, it is then thought to diffuse throughout the body. In addition to its cooling qualities, air is also a kind of *alimento* or food for the body, which provides *fuerza* complementary to that provided by the food one eats.

Sweating is recognized as another means by which the body rids itself of excess heat. The moisture is sometimes said to be the heat itself as it leaves the body. Others explain that the sweating action opens the pores so that cooling air can enter the body. One man describes the moisture as being the strength-giving "juice" obtained from food; thus its loss through sweating explains why one feels weary after hot, exerting work. The absence of sweating in persons with elevated temperatures is taken as indicative of illness, as the excessive heat contained in the body is not being released.

Shivering is explained as a response to cold that has penetrated the body and "reached the heart," and which generates heat through increased activity. Some informants feel that healthy people do not "feel the cold," and thus that shivering is a sign of weakness or sickness.

Sleep and Dreaming

Sleep is considered a necessary and natural state, in which the body rests and the blood builds up *fuerza* to replace that expended during the day's activities. It is viewed as greatly different from unconsciousness: during sleep the mind remains active, whereas in unconsciousness all senses are lost and one is very close to death. Sleep is thought to "heat up" the body, and best occurs at night when the coolness may counteract this tendency. It is considered dangerous to nap during the day and them resume activities, as one risks encountering cold air while still in a heated state. Sleep is viewed as especially important for children, since growth is thought to occur only at this time.

Dreams are the result of the mind's activity while the body is at rest. It is believed that if dreaming did not occur, sleep would be prolonged and one would eventually die. People consistently describe dreams as frightening and disturbing thoughts which serve to awaken one from sleep. People in Pichátaro appear to experience nightmares with some regularity.

THE EXPLANATION OF ILLNESS

In the context of their general views of bodily functioning how do people in Pichátaro explain the occurrence of specific illnesses? We have already mentioned several ways in which illness may occur in relation to particular body parts. Many illnesses, however, are related to more general principles of causation, often to notions of bodily equilibria and how different forces may impinge on them. The organization of our discussion of these principles will anticipate, in part, the distinction between the external versus internal locus of cause to be described in Chapter Four.

Environmental Causes

One of the most frequent and pervasive explanations of how illness occurs is in terms of the pathological effects of agents in the external environment. Cold air, rain, moist ground, the sun, fire, and other features of the environment are commonly believed to be sources of excess heat or cold that may enter the body, upset its normal balance, and cause illness. Excesses of either cold or heat are considered dangerous, especially cold. Illnesses tend to be attributed to cold much more frequently than heat, perhaps due to Pichátaro's predominantly cool, damp climate. Such excesses may be general, or concentrated in a particular part of the body. A common effect of contact with cold is the displacement of the body's normal heat to the head (*calor subido,* or 'risen heat'), where its concentration leads to characteristic symptoms.

The following cases illustrate several features of this theory of temperature equilibrium and the ways in which the balance may be upset. The first is a case of *pulmonía* ('pneumonia'):

> Demetrio had this when he was eighteen years old. It came from the cold. He had gone to La Mojonera [a village in the area] to help with the harvest, and had to sleep on the ground. Later he got wet when he was hot from the work. When he returned home, he began to feel bad. Doña [a curer] made a remedy for him, and he got well with this.

This illness involved a general excess of cold, brought on in two ways. Sleeping on the cool, moist ground caused coldness to enter the body, and getting wet later added to this imbalance. Also evident here is the idea that warm states heighten one's susceptibility to attacks of cold. The next case illustrates an even more common situation involving this notion:

> A while ago my grandmother had *las punzadas* ['sharp headache around the temples']. It came from going right out into the air when she was hot from making tortillas. A current of air hit her. She didn't know how to cure this, so she went to a curer. She got well with this curer's remedies.

At times the interaction of hot and cold forces is more complex, and the specific thermodynamics involved a bit more difficult to work out. Consider this case of *anginas* ('swollen glands in the throat'):

My sister had this last year. It lasted for three days. It came from washing her feet, and then right away coming close to the fire to make tortillas. She got better with a remedy made from roasted tomato and alcohol put on her throat. She also took some pills, and with this she got well. We've always gotten well with this.

Here was a case of "risen heat." The coldness of the water on the girl's feet had the effect of driving her natural body heat upward, creating excesses in the upper part of the body and causing the problem in her throat. The problem was then compounded when this part of her body, already in a state of imbalance, was exposed to even more heat from the kitchen fire and the activity of making tortillas. The treatment involved placing "cool" substances on her throat, which had the effect of neutralizing the excess heat and driving it away from the affected area.

In contrast to the general lack of responsibility for an illness reportedly conceded to the sick person in American society (see Parsons 1951), personal accountability is a more variable matter in Pichátaro, mainly depending upon the ascribed cause of the illness. Those illnesses involving the action of agents in the external environment, as have just been described, are often said to have resulted from a *descuido*—carelessness. These kinds of illnesses are thought preventable if one exercises caution and avoids circumstances which lead to them. To a certain extent, then, a person is considered responsible for what happens as a result of failure to defend against known hazards. In a similar vein, a father may explain that the "cause" of his child's illness was his wife's carelessness in, say, allowing the child to play in a puddle of water. Thus, although Pichatareños do generally view their environment as containing a host of potential threats to their well-being, they do not simply encounter these passively; rather, through awareness, they may often avoid the effects of such hazards.

Internal Causes—Dietary and Emotional

Apart from agents or forces in the external environment which may impinge upon the body's functioning, internally initiated changes in the body's state may also lead to illness. The two principal means by which such internal imbalances are created are one's diet, and strong emotional experiences.

Foods also have "hot" and "cold" qualities,[7] but in a somewhat different sense than when speaking of sources of heat and cold in the external environment. In the latter case, what is involved are actual temperature extremes—cold rain, hot sun, and so on. In the case of foods, however, the "hotness" or "coldness" of a particular item is not dependent upon such a direct reference as temperature. Rather, it is a putative innate quality of the food. For example, pork, mangos, honey, and chilis are considered "hot," while apples, fish, bananas, and potatoes are "cold." All foods ideally have such a quality, although there is a good deal of inconsistency among informants on specific items (see G. Foster 1979). Many items are described as *templado* ('temperate,' or 'medium') and one gets the impression that, for these, the relative "hotness" or "coldness" is not an especially salient characteristic. Nevertheless, there are a number of illnesses that may be brought about due to the particular "hot" or "cold" quality of the foods one eats. This may occur in three different ways.

First, one may simply eat excessive amounts of foods having one or the other quality. One man attributed the diarrhea he was experiencing to the fact that he had recently eaten a lot of honey, which is considered to be very "hot." Similar symptoms may result when excessive amounts of "cold" foods are eaten.

Second, injudicious mixing of items having strongly opposing qualities may cause upsets, as in the following case of *agruras* (a mild stomach ailment):

> Señor _____'s wife had this about four days ago. She had just completed the *cuarentena* ['forty-day period'] after childbirth. She got this because of carelessness: she likes to eat her bread heated, and right after eating some she drank some water. She thinks that this is what made her ill.

We see how the quality of a food may be modified through its method of preparation (here, the bread was made especially "hot"). The bread "heated" her stomach, which made it particularly susceptible to the effects of the "cold" water. The situation was considered compounded by the woman's weakened state following childbirth.

Third, other factors may also predispose the body to harm despite what it ingests. For example, "cold" food and drink, which in normal amounts usually do no harm, may cause illness in a person consuming them while in a highly emotional state. Such states are thought to "heat up" the body.

There are other types of illness closely related to diet, but having nothing to do with the "hot" or "cold" quality of food. Overeating is said to result in a condition known as *empacho* ('blocked digestion'). The person suffering from this is described as literally "stopped up." Unripe fruit is considered especially to cause such a blockage, and this is a frequent illness of children during the time of year when green fruit is available in the orchards. Digestive problems may also be attributed to delays in eating. (The role of the *latido* in these situations has already been described.) Another problem that may occur when eating is delayed too long is that air may enter the empty stomach and create a bloated condition (*sofoca* or *congestión de aire*). At times this condition may be particularly severe, resulting in *cólico* ('colic').

Just as environmentally caused illnesses are said to result from *descuido* ('carelessness'), diet-related illnesses are often ascribed to a *traspaso* ('trespass'). Here, too, is the idea that these illnesses are to some extent within the individual's control and that they are often preventable if one takes care to avoid the circumstances which lead to them. Consider this comment made in reference to a case of *empacho:* "The señor had this about three years ago. 'Just like a child,' says his wife, he was unable to resist eating unripe fruit. She cooked up some herbs for him, and he got well with this." Clearly, the man's wife felt that he should have known better. This is not to say that Pichatareños feel that diet-related illnesses are always avoidable, but rather that the chances of preventing them when proper precautions are taken are sufficient to make the attempt worthwhile.

Another kind of internally initiated imbalance sometimes results from strong emotional experiences. As has been pointed out, Pichatareños believe that intense emotions—such as anger, joy, fright, desire, sorrow, humiliation, and sadness—may result in illness in the person experiencing them. One way in which this occurs is through the "heated" body state such experiences are thought to create. But much more significant are the ways in which strong emotions are thought directly to affect bodily functioning, particularly in relation to the heart, bile, and stomach, but including other parts as well. Here, too, is a kind of bodily balance, although differing somewhat from the idea of the "hot"-"cold" balance, since a concept of specifically opposed qualities is not well developed. Nevertheless, the body does appear to require a moderately steady emotional state. Emotions which are strong enough to upset this equilibrium may lead to illness.

It frequently happens, then, that illness episodes are attributed to strong emotions experienced prior to the onset of the symptoms. The following case of *disentería* ('dysentery'), described by a seventy-year-old man, illustrates this type of explanation:

> I've had it, two days ago—the day before yesterday, and yesterday too. It came from a *sentimiento* ['sorrow'], when my ox died. I had lots of pity—I lost a lot of money. It was like a *bilis*. My wife cooked me a remedy, and with this I got well fast. There was no need to take any pills, or to go to the nuns.

Here, the shock of the animal's death and worry over the loss were considered to have caused the release of "bile" in the body, producing the condition he described as "dysentery." *Bilis* in particular is considered capable of affecting the body in numerous ways, and the symptoms are often quite diffuse. Thus, almost any kind of physical discomfort may have an emotional cause attributed to it, especially when some emotionally upsetting experience has recently occurred.

Emotion-related illnesses are thought to be transferable to small children from their mothers, as in the following instance:

> We had a girl that died of *la bilis*. This happened two years ago. It started when the girl was five months old. Her mother had a *coraje* ['anger'], and then she gave her the breast, and from this the *bilis* started. She was real sick—vomiting and with diarrhea.

Another type of illness commonly believed to be caused by emotions is *enfermedad de corazón* ('heart illness'). It will be recalled that the heart is considered the primary receptor of one's emotional experiences and "pains." Since any feeling of pain, tightness, or uneasiness in the area of the chest is commonly thought to involve the heart, an emotional explanation is usually sought for such problems. One man has thus described his experience:

> Yes, I have this, I'm going along dying of this! When I have feelings of sorrow, my heart begins to hurt. Sometimes my back hurts too, and I start to shake . . . it also starts when I get angry or frightened. . . . I've had this for about a year. At first I took deer's blood, because they say that this is good for it, but this didn't help so my mother told me to go over there to Puácuaro.[8] I didn't have any money, I'm a poor man. . . . I went there to be cured. . . . How good those nurses are. They're Italians, or *gringas,* who knows? They told me to talk to them in Tarasco, and so we talked for a while and they cured me.

One emotion-related illness, *mal de ojo* ('evil eye'), happens in quite a different way. This is an illness specific to children and infants, caused by someone seeing the child and having a strong emotional reaction to it. This is somehow transferred to the child, "irritating the blood," and making it sick. Symptoms include vomiting, diarrhea, general restlessness, and much crying. It is said that anyone may cause this illness, even the child's parents. There are two types of *ojo:* if one has great pleasure and envy upon seeing the child, *ojo de gusto* ('of delight') will result; but if one feels anger, *ojo de coraje* ('of anger') results. The former type is relatively mild and nonserious, the latter severe and potentially fatal. Which form the *ojo* will take is said to depend upon the character of the child's blood. *Ojo de gusto* results if the child has light blood, *ojo de coraje* if its blood is dark and heavy. *Ojo* might equally be considered as a type of illness caused by an external or environmental agent; its place in this scheme is not particularly clear. One man said that *ojo* is caused by "contagion," although, he admitted, of a very special type. As an illness explanation, the *ojo* belief is widespread in Mesoamerica and elsewhere (Adams and Rubel 1967; Maloney

1976; Young 1979b). Its classification in Pichátaro into the two types, however, appears unique.

The idea of personal responsibility, an important feature of the two types of illness explanations previously discussed, is usually absent in emotion-related illnesses. Persons experiencing this type of illness are considered victims of situations which are for the most part beyond their control. Pichatareños tend to view their lives as inevitably entailing times of suffering, disappointment, and interpersonal friction. It follows that what they consider to be a consequence of these experiences—the illnesses described here—also be seen as inevitable. One friend explained *ético,* an illness occurring in children at the time of weaning, thought to result from the loss of motherly affection and jealousy toward the new sibling: "Really it's not an illness, *compadre* . . . it's just a part of life."

Other Explanations of Illness

Thus far discussion has been confined to explanations of what Pichatareños classify as *buena enfermedad* or *enfermedad natural* ('good,' or 'natural illness'). Occasionally, however, illnesses come to be regarded as instances of *mala enfermedad* ('bad illness'), illness caused by witchcraft. It is true that there are people in Pichátaro who engage in malign magic toward others with the intention of causing illness. Most frequently, however, the attribution of a particular illness to witchcraft does not depend upon certain knowledge that someone has indeed instituted it against the victim. Rather, it comes to be suspected in cases which defy treatment.

All cases naming witchcraft as the cause were either chronic and prolonged, or recurrent, illnesses that had repeatedly resisted treatment. Usually such a diagnosis is made by a process of elimination, after home treatment, traditional curers, physicians, and perhaps others have been unsuccessfully tried. Witchcraft then becomes the only reasonable explanation for the persistence of the illness. The attribution of an illness to witchcraft implies a particular kind of treatment. Physicians and others using modern medical remedies are thought unable to cure this type of illness. In these cases either a specialist in curing witchcraft (see Chapter Five), or an acquaintance knowledgeable in these matters, will be consulted. The following case illustrates several features of witchcraft explanations in Pichátaro.

> When José was two years old, he was very sick for about six months. His parents took him to nurses, curers, doctors, "everywhere," without any success in curing him. They thought that he was going to die. One day his father ran into a *compadre* of his, who asked why he looked so sad. The father said that now José was going to die, that there was nothing more to do than to just wait for it. His *compadre* said that he would try to help, and they went and the *compadre* read some cards, all spread out on the table. He concluded that the illness was *mala enfermedad*. The *compadre*'s wife said that she would try to cure José. She gave him a *limpia* (a "brushing," or "cleaning") with a big bunch of leaves and herbs, "of every kind there are here," and continued to give him a *limpia* every morning thereafter for a week. After the week José's father began to notice that he was getting better. At the last *limpia* an egg was also passed over José, and then broken into a glass of water. There they were able to see, in the egg, the illness that had been drawn from him.
>
> His *compadres* refused to take any money for the cure, but in return asked a favor. They were going away to work, and asked José's parents to live in their house and take care of it, and also to care for their orchard. José's parents did so for three years.
>
> The father said that the witchcraft had been aimed at him or his wife, but they were strong and had strong blood and didn't get sick. José, being a child, was not strong enough to resist the illness, but was strong enough to bear it as long as he had it. This is why he did not die.

Here we see how witchcraft was the diagnosis of last resort. As with the cards in this instance, suspicions of witchcraft are usually confirmed through some divinatory procedure. Cases of witchcraft often involve heavy expenses or, as in the above case, incur an obligation which may represent considerable disruption and inconvenience. As an indication of the sensitivity that surrounds the subject of witchcraft, it was not until we had known this family for over eight months of very frequent interaction that they felt willing to relate the case. Up until that time, they had denied any belief in or experience with witchcraft.

Techniques of witchcraft in Pichátaro conform to the classic Frazerian distinction between imitative and contagious magic. One often-mentioned method is to take an image of the intended victim—either a photograph or a doll-like effigy—to one of the caves in the mountains north of town where witchcraft is performed and to leave the image there. The witchcraft may also have its effect when performed on something once in the possession of the victim, as I found in the following instance. Early in the fieldwork, I visited one woman's home in the course of doing the town census. She asked that I give her some money, which I declined to do. Some months later I learned that this woman was one of the town's most famous witches, and related the incident to some friends. I was told that it was a good thing I had not given her anything, as she could have done much harm with it. I was advised not to give things to people with whom I was not well acquainted. Another technique of witchcraft is to place a dangerous substance, such as ground bone from the cemetery, in the victim's food or drink.

Two considerations combine to make witchcraft a relatively infrequent explanation of illness. First, it is rarely suspected in the initial stages of an illness. Second, the vast majority of illnesses in Pichátaro are resolved before reaching the point at which witchcraft represents a plausible explanation, that is, before all routine treatment alternatives have been tried. But in those cases where it is implicated, the consequences for seeking treatment are, as noted above, indeed significant.

Only rarely in Pichátaro does one hear such terms as "contagion" and "microbes" in discussions of illness. These terms refer to concepts having only vague resemblance to the germ theory in Western medicine. Microbes are generally equated with dirtiness, and are said to cause stomach problems and diarrhea when present in one's food. Contagion is most often used to refer to illnesses affecting large numbers of people at the same time. It is sometimes said that these illnesses—such as measles, colds, and whooping cough—are spread from one person to another. But more often, they are explained as due to large numbers of people being exposed to the same environmental conditions that lead to the illness.[9] Overall, very few illnesses in Pichátaro are explained in these terms.

There is the belief in Pichátaro that, in a final sense, illness is something "sent by God" as punishment for one's transgressions. But this belief rarely figures in explanations of particular illnesses, nor is there a specific category of illness said to be "caused by God." Some people interpret "good" or "natural" illness as ultimately "God's will" and "bad" illness (witchcraft-caused) as involving the work of the Devil.

Problems of mechanical origin and those resulting from physical trauma—such as cuts, burns, broken bones, bruises, and sprains— are explained as such, usually without reference to any of the principles of illness causation previously discussed. Such infirmities are commonly said to have resulted from a *descuido* with the same implications for personal responsibility as were discussed earlier.

Prevention

The actions that Pichatareños take in attempting to avoid illness for the most part follow directly from their concepts of the causes of illness. For example, one way to prevent illness believed caused by excess "heat" in the body is to avoid eating large amounts of foods having a "hot" quality. Similarly, people routinely maintain an awareness of external environmental hazards as they go about their daily activities, and they avoid agents such as rain, moist ground, and cold night air, if possible.[10] There are, however, a number of other less obvious practices that deserve mention.

To avoid headaches caused by "attacks" of air when leaving a warm room, many women stick small pieces of a particular kind of leaf on their temples. These are thought to prevent the current from penetrating the head. Similarly, when outdoors at night women pull their *rebozos* ('shawls') tightly around their heads, leaving exposed only the area around the eyes and blocking off cold air that might otherwise enter through the mouth or nose. During warmer weather in April and May, many men schedule their work so that they are idle during the hottest afternoon hours in order to avoid becoming overheated. One man explained his practice of drinking "teas" of *rosa de castilla*—a "fresh" or "cool" herb—during such days, to reduce the risk of heat-induced illness. At any time of the year, people take special precautions when they are hot—either from sickness or from activity—as these are thought to make one particularly susceptible to the harmful effects of cold. People with *calentura* (a "temperature") don't bathe, and men hot from work in the fields allow themselves to "cool off" before washing.

Evil eye may be avoided through the use of several different amulets. The most common is an *ojo de venado* ('deer's eye'), a large seed decorated with beads, red yarn, and a tiny picture of the crucifix, hung around the child's neck on a string. Some mothers prefer to use a small bag containing a few strands of coyote fur, or the feathers of a particular bird. All of these are thought to capture the "evil" and prevent it from harming the child.

Pichatareños believe that the village cemetery is a particularly dangerous place, and they take several precautions relating to it. They claim that one should not go there when sick, nor come in contact with someone who is in a weakened state (such as someone who is ill, or an infant) immediately after visiting it, without first washing away any accumulated dust.

Talking about some types of illness is said occasionally to bring them on, and so people avoid their mention. In particular one should not mention *la fiebre* ('high fever') around someone who is sick with an elevated temperature, as this could worsen the condition. In the same vein, when asked about recent illnesses in the course of the case collection survey, people never reported the absence of illnesses by simply saying "no," but always "no, give thanks to God"—and often several times. They apparently felt the need to ask divine help in keeping illness away from the household.

In addition, Pichatareños have adopted some modern preventive practices. Government vaccination teams visit town several times a year, providing inoculations for whooping cough, diphtheria, tetanus, and polio. While complete data on vaccinations are lacking, it appears that the majority of families have used these services. It seems likely, however, that immunizations that require a series of visits are often not completed, and that periodic revaccinations are often not obtained. People generally believe that vaccinations are valuable and credit them with the present-day absence of small-pox.[11] Some hold the view that vaccinations, especially against whooping cough, do not necessarily prevent their children from getting the illness but do serve to make it milder. Data from a two-day clinic held in November 1975 show that sixty-eight children were vaccinated, over half of them less than a year old. This represents about one-fourth of the total population in that age group.

Illness is thus a matter of considerable and continuing concern to the people of Pichátaro. While sometimes viewed as unpredictable and capricious, once it arrives it must be accounted for and, above all, treated. This section has considered the major causal principles invoked by Pichatareños to explain the occurrence of illness, as well as some of the preventive measures that follow from these principles. However, folk medical knowledge is concerned not only with explaining illness, it is equally concerned with evaluating potential consequences of an illness so that appropriate treatment may be chosen.

EVALUATING THE ILLNESS

An often-assumed model of the illness treatment process is one that proceeds from the initial recognition of symptoms, to the diagnosis or classification of the condition, to the choice and implementation of treatment. For Pichátaro, however, this view that diagnosis is an explicit step in the illness process and must precede decisions about treatment is not necessarily accurate. There is, to be sure, a lexicon of illness terms labeling different diagnostic categories (see Frake 1961). But these terms are often used informally and tentatively in labeling particular illness episodes. There is considerable variation in the implications that a given diagnosis has for the treatment that will be sought. Frequently the specific label used to refer to a condition changes during the course of the illness, reflecting the variable outcomes of different attempts at treatment. The following case is an illustration.

Their one-year-old boy had been sick for about a week with a temperature, cough, runny nose, and had little appetite, a condition which his mother referred to as *gripa* ['cold,' 'flu']. She took him to the nurse in the plaza twice for injections. The last time he had been sick with the *gripa* she had taken him there and he had gotten well. This time, however, he seemed to be getting even sicker—his mother described the illness at this point as "very strong." He was then taken to a "*señora* who knows how to cure" [a folk curer]. The curer said that the problem was really *mollera caída* ['fallen fontanel']. Treatment was given, and the boy began to get well. His mother said that after this she knew why he had not gotten well with the nurse's injections: it was really *la mollera* all along, and this can be cured only with folk remedies.

Two diagnoses are involved here. The first, *gripa,* served primarily as a convenient way of talking about the symptoms. The mother expressed no strong beliefs about what had caused the illness and was willing, with apparently no change in her diagnosis, to consult successively the nurse and a folk curer. The second diagnosis, *mollera caída,* contrasts with the first since it had specific implications both for the cause which was attributed to the illness and for the type of treatment considered appropriate. By definition, this illness is thought caused by a displacement of a section of the top of the skull brought on by a fall, curable only with folk treatment methods. Notice also in this case that the mother's adoption of the diagnosis of *mollera caída* did not precede, but followed from the curer's explanation and seemingly successful treatment of the illness. The latter was strong evidence in support of that diagnosis even though, in this case, the specific symptoms were not those generally associated with *mollera caída.* It is often the case that diagnoses are dependent upon the outcome of treatment.

Like the above example, initial diagnoses of illness in Pichátaro generally describe the symptoms present and usually involve no elaborate diagnostic procedures. If the initial action taken is home treatment, the diagnosis guides selection of an appropriate remedy. However, the initial diagnosis is in most cases too tentative or "loose" to indicate, by itself, the choice of treatment. Subsequent diagnoses, when there are multiple ones, characteristically become increasingly "tight": they point to more specific causes, and sometimes narrow down the range of treatment alternatives considered appropriate. But since the majority of illness episodes in Pichátaro are resolved after the use of only one or two treatment alternatives,[12] and thus do not reach the stage at which such a "tight" diagnosis becomes highly likely, "loose" diagnoses are more often the rule.

Assessing the Gravity of the Illness

What is usually most important to Pichatareños in evaluating symptoms is to determine their seriousness. We developed a card-sorting task in order to investigate how seriousness is classified and how the gravity of particular symptoms is judged. The task involved forty-two different physical and behavioral signs that were known to be of the type people in Pichátaro take as symptomatic of illness. Five literate informants were asked to sort the deck into groups according to how serious they considered the particular symptom. We gave no instructions on how many groups were to be formed. It was explained that the groups should be such that one could consider all the symptoms included in a given group as generally "the same" or "equal" in gravity. We then questioned informants about each symptom and asked why it had been assigned its particular level of gravity.

The same card-sorting task was also done with illness types or diagnostic labels, as opposed to symptoms. The results showed less inter-informant agreement,[13] and a greater number of items went unclassified owing to the opinion that they might vary in gravity, depending upon the particular case and its manifestations. This suggests that in most cases it is not the diagnostic category that primarily determines the seriousness attributed to a given episode, but rather the particular symptoms. Generally, a given symptom has associated with it a much narrower range of judgments about its seriousness than does a given illness label.

We will examine the results of the symptom-ranking task with two questions in mind: 1. In what classes do Pichatareños classify gravity?; and 2. What are the general principles by which particular symptoms are assigned to these classes?

1. The results suggest that in Pichátaro the seriousness of an illness is generally thought of in terms of three basic levels. Illnesses of the first level are described as 'little' *(chica)*, 'brief' *(corta)*, or 'simple' *(sencilla)*; the second level, 'regular' *(regular)*, 'medium' *(mediana)*, or 'more complicated' *(más complicada)*; and the third level, 'grave' *(grave)*, 'dangerous' *(peligrosa)*, or 'heavy' *(pesada)*. For present purposes, these three classes will be referred to simply as nonserious, moderately serious, and grave. We must keep in mind that these are not arbitrary or analytic distinctions, but rather reflect how gravity was classified by this group of informants.

In the actual task, three informants formed three groups, and two formed four. Each of the groups had varying numbers of symptoms included in them. The latter two cases, where four groups were formed, both split the initial grave category into two sets. Both sets indicated potentially fatal conditions—the key attribute of the grave class. The informants generally agreed that the treatment implications would be the same for both sets. Therefore, we can assume that a three-level model of seriousness is generally representative of the magnitudes of difference that have significance for treatment decisions.

The content of the three levels is illustrated in Table 3.1. Symptoms[14] are listed according to the class in which they were most frequently placed by informants (the modal category). For each symptom, the median rank is indicated.

Agreement on the particular symptoms included in the categories was not exceptionally high (average $r_s = 0.55$).[15] Thus, if the purpose of the study had been to arrive at a generally valid seriousness rating for each specific symptom, there might be some cause to question the usefulness of the results. This was not, however, the purpose; rather, it was to observe the number of classes employed by informants in judging illness gravity and the principles by which particular symptoms were assigned to these classes. No attempt will be made in the course of later analysis to assign a level of gravity to particular illness occurrences on the basis of the symptoms reported. Instead, in those situations where seriousness ratings of specific illnesses are required—and they are quite important in the

Table 3.1. **Composite Sorting with Median Seriousness Ratings for Each Symptom**

Nonserious		Moderately serious		Grave	
7.8	headache	19.5	body aches	32.4	swollen glands
8.0	sticky eye	20.0	not being able to		in the throat
	discharge		go to the bathroom	34.0	difficulty breathing
8.0	runny nose	20.5	aching in the bones	34.0	vomiting
9.0	pimples on skin	21.0	red spots on skin	34.0	unconsciousness
9.0	sore throat	23.5	not being able to eat	36.0	high fever
9.0	sleeplessness	24.5	diarrhea	37.5	heavy bleeding
9.0	motion sickness	24.5	aching in back	37.5	pains in the heart
9.0	body feels cold	24.5	bloody stool		
9.5	toothache	24.5	bleeding from nose		
10.0	weakness	24.5	pains in the chest		
10.9	aching joints	24.5	colic pains		
10.9	chills	25.7	earache		
10.9	stomachache	26.9	coughing up phlegm		
10.9	nervousness	27.1	swelling		
10.9	dizziness	27.8	stretched veins		
10.9	lack of appetite		and nerves		
		27.8	unable to walk		

model of treatment choice described in Chapter Six—it is the level of gravity perceived and reported by the informant that is employed. What we need some assurance of, then, is that when informants describe an illness as *chica* or *peligrosa,* these terms refer to a relatively stable and shared scheme of gravity classification. This assurance is provided by the fact that in the present study, although the content of the classes sometimes varied, their basic structure remained quite constant; informants invariably formed a small, and usually like, number of gravity classes and described these classes in much the same ways.

2. What are the general principles used to assign particular symptoms to these classes? Perhaps most salient is whether or not the symptoms indicate a potential or direct threat to life. It was frequently apparent that informants were using the following sorting criterion: nonserious symptoms clearly do not threaten life. Moderately serious symptoms similarly do not indicate a life-threatening condition, but such symptoms on occasion have been precursors of conditions that were ultimately fatal. Grave symptoms represent

conditions that may directly result in the victim's death. The following excerpts from one interview illustrate this reasoning and also point out some other considerations involved in judging the seriousness of an illness.

Nonserious (sore throat)

Q Sometimes people say that they have . . . a sore throat. Does this indicate much gravity?

A This is also . . . just a passing thing. One keeps going on with this. Maybe others . . . but us, we just keep going when we have this. Sometimes it's just because you drink cold water when you're warm . . . it goes here [indicates first level].

Moderately serious (not being able to eat)

Q Sometimes people say that they're not able to eat, that they just can't eat anything. Is this a thing of much gravity, or not so much?

A Yes, sometimes you just don't have any desire to eat, and other times, you eat something, and just throw it up. It just doesn't agree with you—you can't take it.

Q So when it's like this, is that regular, or grave, or just a little thing, or what?

A Yes, it's, well, serious . . . I mean you're sick all right . . . it's natural for us here . . . it's something that keeps advancing, advancing. One doesn't die of this, but by and by it's advancing . . . it's debilitating the person.

Q Then does it go here [indicating third level] or here [indicating second level]?

A I think here [indicating second level].

Grave (pains in the heart)

Q Sometimes people have heart pains, pains right in the heart. Does this indicate much gravity?

A Always, yes . . . by all means, yes. It's inside, really inside. I mean, it's the heart!

In judging the seriousness of an illness, Pichatareños also consider the degree of incapacitation. As in the case of the symptom "sore throat," the fact that one "keeps on going" and does not re-

main in bed[16] or forgo normal activities usually goes along with a
judgment of nonseriousness. Moderately serious symptoms, on the
other hand, usually do involve a curtailment of normal activities;
routinely the victim remains in bed and observes dietary restrictions. Conditions judged grave, as one might expect, always involve
a complete suspension of activities.

Elevated body temperature occurs with many illnesses, and
Pichatareños regard it as a direct indicator of the extent of the hot-
cold imbalance in the body. Two symptoms included in the card-
sorting task related to temperature: *calentura* and *fiebre*. Both
terms may be translated as 'fever,' but *fiebre* by definition indicates
an extreme fever, and all informants considered it grave. (*Fiebre* is
listed as 'high fever' in Table 3.1.) In rating the symptom *calentura*,
however, all five informants explained that its seriousness would
depend upon how high the fever is. When fever does occur, then, the
gravity attributed to the illness is almost always directly related to
the degree of heat detected, and may range from nonserious to
grave.[17]

The extent to which a given symptom is thought to interfere with
a vital bodily part or process is also significant in these judgments.
Thus breathing difficulty is grave, as are severe vomiting[18] (inter-
feres with the provision of *fuerza*), and heart pains and bleeding
(interfere with the distribution of *fuerza*). The reason that Pichatareños regard some symptoms, which the observer might initially
consider nonserious (such as backache) as moderately serious becomes clear when we understand what the symptoms represent in
terms of the local view of bodily structure and function.

The gravity which will be attributed to a condition involving
pain is directly related to the level of discomfort. The locus of pain
is especially relevant. Pains located deep inside the body (see above,
"pains in the heart") are considered more serious than those occurring at the surface or in the extremities. Most surface symptoms are
regarded as nonserious, since they are unlikely to indicate interfer-
ence with important parts. Thus common eye problems and skin
disorders are nonserious, unless they are judged to indicate a
deeper-lying dysfunction (such as "red spots on skin," which indicates excessive heat within the body).

THE DISTRIBUTION OF TYPES
OF ILLNESS

The system of folk medical knowledge described here should be viewed within the context of what constitutes a typical occurrence of illness in Pichátaro. With what frequencies, then, do Pichatareños invoke the different principles of illness causation and evaluation when illness strikes? Data on this issue come from a set of illness case histories collected from a representative sample of Pichátaro households. Over a six-month period, sixty-two households were visited on an approximate biweekly basis and records made of each illness occurring among its members (details of the case collection procedures are given in Appendix A). These data were collected primarily to obtain a body of independent cases with which to test the model of treatment decision making (see Chapter Six), but they may also serve to provide a summary view of the incidence of illness in Pichátaro.

Table 3.2 lists the twenty most frequent illness types among the 323 cases recorded. In those instances where the diagnostic label used to refer to the condition changed in the course of the illness, only the ultimate diagnosis is included. In all cases, these represent the informants' designation of the illness. Most of the types listed have either been described elsewhere in this chapter or are largely self-explanatory; while a detailed explanation of each therefore seems unnecessary here, a few comments are in order. *Calentura* is generally used to designate *gripa*-like conditions which are mild and involve primarily an elevated temperature. *Diarrea,* or *deposiciones,* is a milder form of intestinal upset than *disentería;* the latter diagnosis depends upon the presence of blood in the stool. *Anginas* may stem from excess heat in the upper part of the body, and may also result from "not crying when you feel like it." *Punzadas* involves sharp pains around the temples or in the inner ear, which are thought caused by "airs" which have penetrated the head. *Fogazo* is a general condition of excess heat in the body, and commonly breaks out in the form of sores on the lips. *Tos ferina* is an illness "of a term"—it is thought to last forty days, and affects only children.

Table 3.2. **The Twenty Most Frequent Illness Types in the Case Collection Sample**

Type and English gloss	Percentage of total cases
Gripa ('cold,' 'flu')	22.9
Calentura (a 'temperature')	9.6
Empacho ('blocked digestion')	4.6
Diarrea, deposiciones ('diarrhea')	4.6
Anginas ('swollen glands in the neck')	3.7
Bilis ('bile')	3.7
Sofoca del estómago ('bloated stomach')	3.1
Calor subido ('risen heat')	2.8
Muelas ('toothache')	2.5
Punzadas ('sharp headache around temples')	2.5
Enfermedad de corazón ('heart illness')	2.2
Disentería ('dysentery')	2.2
Cólico ('colic')	2.2
Vómito ('vomiting')	2.2
Herida ('wound')	2.2
Latido ('palpitations')	1.9
Fogazo ('fever sores')	1.9
Sarampión ('measles')	1.6
Tos ferina ('whooping cough')	1.6
Mal de ojo ('evil eye')	1.6

The most common illnesses in Pichátaro are *gripa* and *calentura,* which together represent almost one-third of all cases in the sample. Included within this category, however, are conditions involving varying levels of gravity and resulting in a variety of choices of treatment. The remaining two-thirds include a wide range of illness types: in the complete set of 323 episodes, in fact, over sixty different diagnoses are represented. The ascribed cause of nearly 40% of the cases involved external environmental agents, the most frequently named being "the cold" and "airs." Around 20% of the cases were attributed to dietary causes, and almost 10% to emotional causes. For a good number of the remaining cases, informants said that they did not know the cause or were not sure of it. Over half (54%) of the cases were judged to be nonserious, one-third were judged at some point to be moderately serious, and around 15% were considered grave. A third of all the cases involved victims less than five years of age—about twice that expected on the basis of the proportion of individuals of that age group in the total population. Illnesses were reported for the remaining age groups in proportion to or below their representation in the population, with the exception of the thirty-five to fifty-year age group, which is overrepresented by about 40%. Fewer cases were reported for males than for females, although the difference is not great. In duration, 30% of the illnesses lasted three days or less, 46% persisted for between four days and a week, around 12% for one to two weeks; the remaining 12% lasted for over two weeks. (Data on the treatment choices to which these cases led are summarized in Chapter Six.)

Thus far, a primarily descriptive approach has been taken in our treatment of the Pichátaro system of folk medical knowledge. The next chapter adopts a more formal perspective on this system. We will consider a set of beliefs about illness and a set of terms used to describe different illnesses, employing a procedure that allows us to discover the more inclusive categories of illness inherent in these data. Examination of the features distinguishing these categories yields useful insights into the general principles of categorization and also suggests some of the links between what people in Pichátaro believe to be true about illness and the actions they take in response to it.

4

The Structuring of Folk
Medical Knowledge

When people think about alternative actions for dealing with a particular problem, they naturally often consider past actions in similar situations. We can assume that people with a particular illness will do the same. Classifications of illness then come to be structured in terms of distinctions that are preparatory to action. Determination of these distinctions is one way of gaining insight into the relationship between medical beliefs and behavior relating to illness. My intention in this chapter is to discover these distinctions by formally analyzing a classification of illness types in Pichátaro.

For many Mesoamerican communities the distinction separating illnesses which are caused by excess "heat" from illnesses caused by excess "cold" (see Chapter Three) has long been considered to be a primary element in the classification of illness. In contrast, the present analysis shows the "hot"-"cold" distinction to have considerably less importance than certain other distinctions in accounting for the categories of illness present in the data.

THE ILLNESS BELIEF DATA

The data examined here are from a standardized interview that was developed and carried out as follows:[1] initially a number of informants were interviewed concerning illness beliefs and practices by use of frame questioning techniques (see Metzger and Williams 1963) and open-ended questioning. These interviews provided statements about illness that were then recast in the form of question frames. The result was a large set of frames that involved a variety of concerns and beliefs about illness as it is locally understood, including causes, cures, situations leading to illness, symptoms, consequences, gravity, and types of victim. The frames are representative of the interests that lay people express when they talk about illness. All illness terms that appeared in the interviews were also compiled, and with the advice of two informants, I eliminated unfamiliar or ambiguous terms. I then constructed a preliminary question matrix and pretested it with three informants. Frames that these informants found difficult to interpret or that allowed disparate interpretations were removed. The revised question matrix was then administered to ten informants (six women and four men), representing a range of occupations and ages. The interview was lengthy (over two thousand questions), and so each informant was questioned in approximately hour-long sessions occurring over several days. In the interview, each illness term was paired with each question frame, and the informant was asked to reply as to whether she (or he) agreed that the particular attribute contained in the question applied to the given illness.

Results of the interviews were combined by recording as a "yes" all attribute-term pairs for which the majority of informants (six or more) responded affirmatively.[2] Several attributes that had low variance across illness types (applying to nearly all or very few) were removed at this point, and the final result was a 43 (attribute) × 34 (term) data matrix, in which each cell contains an X ("yes") or is blank ("no") (Table 4.1).

Table 4.2 gives the question frames and their approximate English translations. The word(s) italicized in each frame appears on the data matrix. Similarly, Table 4.3 lists illness terms along with their English glosses. The English terms are not equivalent to the Spanish, but serve to summarize in a general way the nature of the illnesses involved. As will be apparent, the terms and attributes considered here are by no means exhaustive of Pichatareño illness beliefs—rather, they are presented as a generally representative sample of them.

Table 4.1. **Data Matrix**

```
                                                                            N
                 K                                                          O
                 N                                                          T
                 O                               C                          
                 C                               A                 S        B
                 K    C                     B    R         F       T   N    A
                 S  H C  B  D          B    A    E     G   R       M   O    A  T
                    I H  O  R          A    T    L     H   R   M   U   U    S  H
                 F  H O  L  E          T    H    E     R   I   M   S   S    I  N
                 A  O U  S  N          H    W    V     A   G   U   A   E    E  G
                 L  U L  S  E          W    E    A     V   A   S   C        N  
                 L  T T  S  S          E         T     E   T   H   H
              ─────────────────────────────────────────────────────────────────
Pneumonia           X  X  X  X            X    X  X  X       X       X           X
Bloated Stomach     X                      X                             X
Measles             X  X                                     X
Smallpox            X                                        X
Witchcraft          X  X  X  X                               X           X  X
Swollen Glands      X                           X  X  X
Heart Illness       X     X                                  X  X
Dysentery                       X                      X  X          X
Toothache              X                                     X
Grippe           X  X  X  X  X  X       X  X  X  X  X  X       X       X  X
Bronchopneumonia X  X     X             X  X  X  X       X       X
Embolio          X  X             X  X                   X   X  X          X
Whooping Cough            X                             X  X                    X
Mollera Caída    X                                      X  X
Sharp Headache      X     X             X  X  X  X  X       X
Colic               X  X                X                X  X       X
Itchy Rash                                                                      X
Sprains and Bruises X X  X  X           X  X                 X
Acid Stomach                           X                                X
Temperature      X  X  X  X       X  X  X  X  X  X  X       X       X  X
Blocked Digestion                      X                 X       X       X
Rheumatism          X                   X  X  X  X  X
Bile             X        X                             X  X       X
Motion Sickness                                 X                            X
Attacks             X                                  X  X                  X
Asthma                    X                             X
Palpitations        X                   X              X           X
Evil Eye
Fever Sores            X                X  X                 X                  X
Fever            X  X  X          X  X  X  X  X  X  X       X       X  X
Relapse          X  X  X  X  X  X  X  X  X          X       X
Bronchitis       X  X  X  X             X  X  X          X       X
Vomiting         X  X  X          X                X       X  X       X  X
Risen Heat                             X  X  X  X
```

```
    T C
    E O
    M L                    C                          N
  A P D   C       C        O              S           O
  P E       O B     H    N W            C P           T            V
  P R T P L R       A    T E G    A     H R           E            O
  E P A H H D E A N      A A R C D      I L I D       E            M
  T I T I L   A N G      G T O O U H C D T K C C T    B W          I
  I L U N E A T G I O I  H U U L E O R T L T O I O    E I          T
  T L R G G I H E N L O  E N G T A O E L E O L N D    A N          I
  E S E S M R E R G D N  R D H S D L N E S R D G Y    K G          N
  ────────────────────────────────────────────────────────────────
  X X X    X X X   X X   X X X              X X X   X
  X X   X     X                        X        X X              X
  X   X              X X            X       X X     X X
  X   X              X X            X                       X X X
  X         X   X       X             X                 X X X
  X X X    X X X         X           X      X X X       X
              X X     X           X   X         X       X
  X X   X               X               X
  X X     X                       X X   X   X   X
  X X X     X       X X X X X X     X       X X X     X X X
  X X X X X X X     X X     X X           X X X       X
  X         X X   X   X         X          X   X X
              X   X   X   X X     X   X       X X
      X                       X   X X             X
  X X       X X       X X       X         X X X     X
  X       X       X   X         X         X X X     X
                  X X       X     X   X     X

      X   X                       X             X
  X X X     X     X X X X X X       X       X X X X   X X X
  X X   X                         X           X       X X
        X             X   X           X X X
  X            X             X X X             X X
  X X               X         X X   X       X     X X
        X       X X               X       X   X X
              X           X X   X         X     X X
  X                       X             X           X X
                              X X         X X
                    X         X X         X X
  X X X     X     X X X X X X     X       X X     X X X
  X   X     X     X X       X X   X       X X X     X X
  X X X     X       X X     X             X X       X
  X X     X X   X X   X             X       X X X X X X
        X               X       X         X X   X X
```

Table 4.2. **Question Frames**

1. ¿Viene _____ por una *caída*? (Does _____ come from a *fall*?)

2. ¿Cuando uno tiene _____ , tiene que tomar cosas *calientes* para curarse? (When one has _____ , does one have to take *"hot"* things to be cured?)

3. ¿Se *cae* uno cuando tiene _____ ? (Does it *"knock* you *out"* when one has _____ ?)

4. ¿Hay *escalofrío* con _____ ? (Are there *chills* with _____ ?)

5. ¿Hay dolores en el *pecho* con _____ ? (Are there pains in the *chest* with _____ ?)

6. ¿Duelen los *huesos* con _____ ? (Do the *bones* ache with _____ ?)

7. ¿Puede venir _____ por una *borrachera*? (Can _____ come from a *"drunk"*?)

8. ¿Cuando uno tiene calentura y se *baña,* se puede agarrar _____ ? (When one has a "temperature" and *bathes,* can one catch _____ ?)

9. ¿Cuando se *moja* uno, se puede agarrar _____ ? (When one gets *wet,* can one catch _____ ?)

10. ¿Viene _____ por *descuido*? (Does _____ come from *careless*ness?)

11. ¿Viene _____ por el *calor*? (Does _____ come from the *"heat"*?)

12. ¿Es _____ una enfermedad *grave*? (Is _____ a *grave* illness?)

13. ¿Puede venir _____ por un *susto*? (Can _____ come from a *fright*?)

14. ¿Viene _____ por un *aire*? (Does _____ come from an *"air"*?)

15. ¿Con _____ hay dolor en el *estómago*? (With _____ is there pain in the *stomach*?)

16. ¿Con _____ hay un *mareo*? (With _____ is there *nausea*?)

17. ¿Proviene _____ por *no bañarse* ni cambiar la ropa? (Does _____ come from *not bathing* or changing your clothes?)

18. ¿Cuando tiene _____ no tiene *hambre*? (Do you not have an *appetite* with _____ ?)

19. ¿Puede curar _____ con *pastillas*? (Can you cure _____ with *pills*?)

20. ¿Con _____ hay *calentura*? (With _____ is there a *"temperature"*?)

21. ¿Se puede agarrar _____ por comer muchas *cosas frescas*? (Can you get _____ from eating a lot of *"cold" things*?)

22. ¿Con _____ sale saliva espesa, *flema*? (With _____ does *phlegm* come up?)

23. ¿Cuando sale de un lugar caliente y entra en el *aire frío,* se puede agarrar _____ ? (When you leave a warm place and enter into the *cold air,* can you catch _____ ?)

24. ¿Cuando uno tiene _____ , no puede *respirar* bien? (When one has _____ , can one not *breathe* well?)

25. ¿Puede venir _____ por un *coraje*? (Can _____ come from *anger*?)

26. ¿Se agarra mucho aquí _____ cuando está *cambiando* el tiempo? (Do they catch _____ a lot here when the weather is *changing*?)

27. ¿No resisten bien _____ gente con *muchos años*? (Do *old* people not resist _____ well?)

28. ¿Viene _____ por *contagio* de otras personas? (Does _____ come from *contagion* from other people?)

29. ¿Viene _____ en el *tiempo* de calor? (Does _____ come in hot *weather*?)

30. ¿Viene _____ por reposar en el *suelo*? (Does _____ come from laying on the *ground*?)

31. ¿Con _____ hay *tos*? (With _____ is there a *cough*?)

32. ¿Es _____ una enfermedad solamente de *gente grande*? (Is _____ an illness of just *adults*?)

33. ¿Con _____ duele la *cabeza*? (With _____ does the *head* hurt?)

34. ¿Cuando uno tiene _____ , tiene que tomar cosas *frescas* para curarse? (When you have _____ , do you have to take "*cool*" things to be cured?)

35. ¿Es _____ una enfermedad solamente de los *niños*? (Is _____ an illness of only *children*?)

36. ¿Es _____ una enfermedad *corta,* no muy grave? (Is _____ a *little* illness, not very serious?)

37. ¿Se agarra mucho _____ cuando cae la *aguita*? (Do they catch _____ a lot when it "*sprinkles*"?)

38. ¿Con _____ tiene que ir al *doctor*? (With _____ do you have to go to the *doctor*?)

39. ¿Sobreviene _____ por el *frío*? (Does _____ come from the *cold*?)

40. ¿Viene _____ por *no comer* a las horas? (Does _____ come from *not eating* at the right times?)

41. ¿Con _____ duele todo el *cuerpo*? (With _____ does the whole *body* ache?)

42. ¿Se pone uno *debilitado* cuando tiene _____ ? (Does it make you *weak* when you have _____ ?)

43. ¿Con _____ hay *vómito*? (With _____ is there *vomiting*?)

_____

Note: Spanish frames reflect local usage.

Table 4.3. **Illness Terms**

1.	*Pulmonía*	pneumonia
2.	*Sofoca del estómago*	bloated stomach
3.	*Sarampión*	measles
4.	*Viruela*	smallpox
5.	*Enfermedad de brujería*	witchcraft-caused illness
6.	*Anginas*	swollen glands in the neck
7.	*Enfermedad de corazón*	heart illness
8.	*Disentería*	dysentery
9.	*Muelas*	toothache
10.	*Gripa*	grippe (cold, flu)
11.	*Broncomonía*	bronchopneumonia
12.	*Embolio*	a sudden grave attack that knocks the victim unconscious
13.	*Tos ferina*	whooping cough
14.	*Mollera caída*	displacement of a section of the top of the skull
15.	*Punzadas*	sharp headache around the temples
16.	*Cólico*	colic, sharp stomach pains
17.	*Sarna*	itchy rash
18.	*Lastimadura*	sprains, strains, bruises
19.	*Agruras*	acid stomach
20.	*Calentura*	a temperature, mild fever
21.	*Empacho*	blocked digestion
22.	*Reumatismo*	rheumatism
23.	*Bilis*	bile, illness resulting from strong emotions
24.	*Almareos*	motion sickness
25.	*Ataques*	attacks
26.	*Asma*	asthma
27.	*Latido*	palpitations
28.	*Mal de ojo*	evil eye
29.	*Fogazo*	fever sores
30.	*Fiebre*	fever
31.	*Desmando, recaída*	relapse
32.	*Bronquitis*	bronchitis
33.	*Vómito*	vomiting
34.	*Calor subido*	risen heat

CLUSTER ANALYSIS

All of the data are shown in Table 4.1, but in this form the categorical structuring of the data and the relationships among illness types and their attributes are difficult to assess. I used cluster analysis to reveal these features.

Cluster analysis refers to a number of related statistical classification techniques that take data units (in this case, illness terms or illness attributes) and, ideally, group them into clusters so that "elements within a cluster have a high degree of 'natural association' among themselves while the clusters are 'relatively distinct' from one another" (Anderberg 1973:xi). The extent to which a procedure results in such clusters depends upon the structuring inherent in the data. Hierarchical clustering techniques produce representations of the data units that are analogous to the taxonomies of descriptive semantics (Burton 1972:560) and can be presented in the form of tree diagrams.

The basis of categorization is judged similarity, and here similarity is defined in terms of the sharing of attributes. I constructed a matrix of similarity measures for all possible illness-illness and attribute-attribute pairs on the basis of the number of attributes the two members of each pair have in common. In concrete terms, the measure reflects similarity in the patterning of Xs and blanks for each pair of items in the data matrix. Each time two items share the same attribute or both lack it counts as one unit in determining the similarity score for that pair.[3]

The clustering procedure used is based on Johnson's hierarchical clustering method (1967). This procedure takes as input the matrix of similarity measures for all possible item pairs and produces a tree diagram in which any two items are joined in a cluster at the level of their similarity. Figures 4.1 and 4.2 present the results of the clustering of the illness terms and illness attributes and reveal a significant structuring of the data. The scale running across the top of each diagram represents the percentage of attributes shared. (In Figure 4.2 the illness terms become the "attributes.") Highly similar items (for example, grippe and temperature in Figure 4.1) are grouped low (toward the right) in the diagram, whereas items with low similarities are included in the same cluster only at high (toward the left) levels. The result is a graphic representation of the data that readily lends itself to interpretation.[4]

If we examine the illness terms (Figure 4.1), the first major division (between clusters I and II) appears to be between cold-like and respiratory illnesses, and all other types. Cluster II then appears to divide generally between illnesses affecting the stomach and gut, and all others. Altogether nine clusters are distinguished within major clusters I and II, including two (rheumatism and whooping cough) that consist of a single illness type. I arrived at the nine

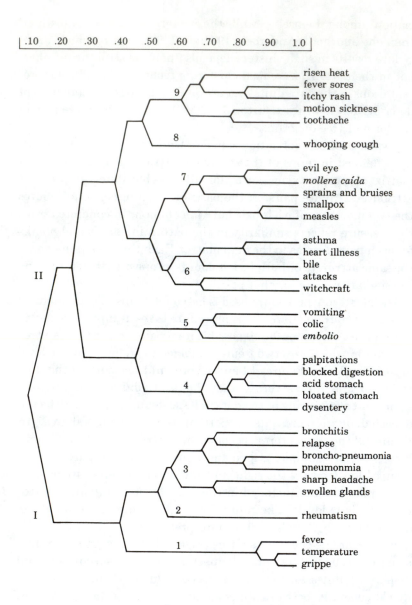

Figure 4.1. **Hierarchical Clustering of Illness Terms**

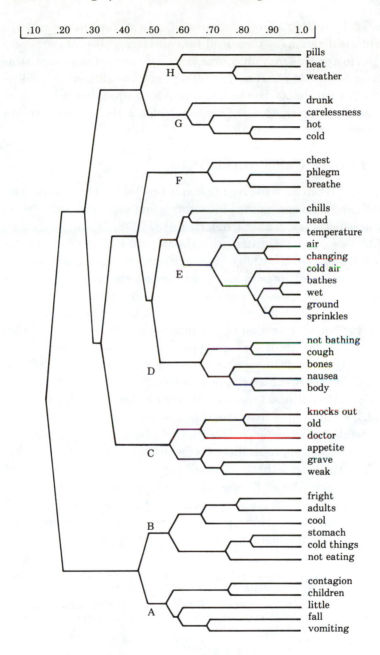

Figure 4.2. **Hierarchical Clustering of Illness Attributes**

clusters by setting a level of approximately .60 (on the scale at the top of the diagram) as the cutoff for considering a set of terms as a single cluster. One may, of course, consider the results as consisting of from one to 34 clusters, depending upon the clustering level selected. I used the .60 level since it provided what seemed the best balance between the goals of achieving high within-cluster and low between-cluster similarity.

ATTRIBUTE CRITERIALITY

Our interpretation of the results is aided by taking the original data matrix and rearranging the illness terms and attributes into the order in which they cluster (Anderberg 1973:178; D'Andrade, et al., 1972). This gives the distributional patterning of the data (Table 4.4) and aids identification of the attributes of a given illness cluster. For example, illnesses in cluster 7 are associated, in varying degrees, with "hot" weather, chills, not coming from an "air," "temperature," gravity, children, and so on. What may become apparent upon further examination of the distributional patterning is that some attributes are more significant than others in their relative exclusivity to that illness cluster. Consider, for example, the relationship between the attribute *children* ("an illness only of children") and the illness types included in cluster 7, tabulated in Figure 4.3. In four out of five cases illnesses with the attribute *children* are members of cluster 7. In other words, possession of this attribute affects the probability of a given illness term falling in cluster 7, to the extent that 80% of all terms having it are in fact included. To consider all illnesses, however, and not just those having the given attribute, it is also necessary to take into account the proportion of illnesses within a given cluster that actually possess that attribute. A simple measure called "criteriality" may be defined as follows:[5]

$$
\begin{array}{l}
\text{criteriality of} \\
\text{attribute } x \text{ for} \\
\text{a given cluster}
\end{array}
=
\frac{
\begin{array}{l}
\text{number of illnesses with} \\
\text{attribute } x \text{ in cluster}
\end{array}
}{
\begin{array}{l}
\text{total number of illnesses} \\
\text{with attribute } x
\end{array}
}
\times
\frac{
\begin{array}{l}
\text{number of illnesses with} \\
\text{attribute } x \text{ in cluster}
\end{array}
}{
\begin{array}{l}
\text{total number of illnesses} \\
\text{included in cluster}
\end{array}
}
$$

$$
= \frac{a^2}{(a + b)(a + c)}
$$

This gives a measure of the importance of a given attribute in accounting for cluster membership. For example, an attribute with a criteriality of 1.0 for a given cluster would be possessed by all illnesses included in that cluster and no others; an attribute of 0 criteriality would be possessed by none of the illnesses in that cluster. Analysis in terms of criteriality distinguishes those attributes that are characteristic of particular clusters from those that are more general.

As an illustration, Table 4.5 shows the criteriality of all attributes that apply to one or more illnesses included in cluster 7. It is clear that what is primarily characteristic of the set of illnesses in this cluster is their restriction to children.

Analysis in this fashion of the entire set of reordered data reveals that a relatively small number of highly criterial attributes may be isolated.[6] The first step in this analysis was to consider the two major clusters (labeled I and II in Figure 4.1) and determine the most highly criterial attribute distinguishing these two groupings. Then, I determined, progressively, the most highly criterial attribute at the next node (where cluster 1 splits from 2 and 3), and finally, the most highly criterial attribute distinguishing clusters 2 and 3. The same procedure was followed for cluster II. At each stage I calculated criteriality by considering the distribution of the attribute only across the illnesses joined at that node. In only the first instance, then, did I determine criteriality across the entire set of illness terms, since this is the only node at which the entire set is joined. In each case, the highly criterial attribute reflects the principal contrast between those adjacent clusters. Figure 4.4 gives the results by superimposing over an outline of the illness tree diagram the attribute found to be most highly criterial at each node. I have indicated the criteriality of the attribute for the clusters joined at that node.

To assess the model's descriptive adequacy, I passed each illness type through the chart and checked for the presence or absence of each attribute encountered in its path. Of the thirty-four terms, twenty-nine (85%) were correctly placed. For the data in general, then, it appears that these highly criterial attributes do represent important kinds of distinctions for comprehending the categories.

Table 4.4. **Distributional Patterning for Hierarchical Clustering**

Illness	PILLS	WEATHER	CARDEHER	DRUNK	CHILLS	COUGH	PHLEGM	CHEST	WITCHCRAFT	BILE	HEART	RELAPSE	CHILLS	HEAT	TEMPERATURE	CHANGE	COLD	BATHS
Grippe	X	X	X	X	X	X	X	X				X	X	X	X	X	X	X
Temperature	X	X	X	X	X	X						X	X	X	X	X	X	X
Fever	X	X	X	X	X	X						X	X	X	X	X	X	X
Rheumatism				X	X	X	X										X	X
Swollen Glands	X				X		X		X	X		X	X	X			X	X
Sharp Headache	X	X	X		X	X				X		X	X		X		X	X
Pneumonia	X		X	X	X	X	X	X	X	X	X	X		X	X	X	X	X
Bronchopneumonia	X		X	X	X	X	X	X	X	X	X			X	X	X	X	X
Relapse				X	X	X	X	X				X	X	X	X	X	X	
Bronchitis	X		X		X	X	X	X				X		X	X	X	X	X
Dysentery	X	X	X	X														
Bloated Stomach	X			X		X	X			X								
Acid Stomach	X			X														
Blocked Digestion	X				X													
Palpitations				X	X	X												
Embolio				X	X	X		X									X	
Colic				X		X	X											
Vomiting	X			X	X	X	X			X	X							
Witchcraft								X	X	X	X	X	X					
Attacks	X									X		X						
Bile												X	X					
Heart Illness								X		X		X						
Asthma								X										
Measles		X										X		X				
Smallpox		X										X		X				
Sprains and Bruises				X	X	X						X						
Mollera Caída				X									X	X				
Evil Eye																		
Whooping Cough		X	X					X	X	X	X		X					
Toothache	X	X								X	X			X				
Motion Sickness	X	X	X									X						
Itchy Rash		X																
Fever Sores		X	X	X								X						X
Risen Heat		X	X		X								X	X				X

```
        N                                         C
        O                                         O   N
    S   T                   K                     L   O   C
    P                       N           A         D   T   O   C               C
    R   B                   O           P      S      N   H           V       L
G   I   A       N           K       D   P   F  A   T  T   E   T   I   L   M    S
R   N   T   C   B   A       S       O   E   G  R  D   O   H   A   A   L   I    I   T
O   K   H   O   O   U   B           C   T   R  W  I  U   C   M   I   T   G   D  T   F   T   E
W   U   L   I   U   N   S   O   O   O   T   I  A  E  G   L   O   A   N   I   I  R   T   A   I   R
E   N   E   N   G   E   E   D   U   L   O   T  V  A  H   T   O   C   G   N   O  E   L   L   N
T   D   S   G   H   S   A   Y   T   D   R   E  E  K  T   S   L   H   S   G   N  N   E   L   G   #
```

```
X X X │ X X X X X │ X X X X X X │           │ X     X X X
X X X │ X X X X X │ X X X X X X │           │ X     X X X   1
X X X │ X X X X X │ X X X X X X │           │ X       X
─────────────────────────────────────────────────────────
X X X │     X     │     X       │   X       │               2
─────────────────────────────────────────────────────────
      │           │ X X     X   │           │
X X   │           │ X X X X     │         X │
X X X │ X X     X │ X X X X X   │           │               3
X X X │           │ X X X X   X │           │
X X X │     X X   │ X X X X X X │           │
X     │           │ X X X X X X │           │
─────────────────────────────────────────────────────────
      │           │       X X   │   X X X   │
      │         X │       X     │   X X X   │ X     X
      │           │             │   X X X   │ X       4
      │         X │     X X X   │   X X X   │ X     X
      │           │       X X   │ X X   X   │           X
─────────────────────────────────────────────────────────
      │     X X X │ X     X X X X │ X X       │
      │           │ X X   X X X │ X     X X X │             5
      │     X X   │ X X X X X X X │ X   X X X X │     X X
─────────────────────────────────────────────────────────
      │     X X X │ X X   X X X │   X         │         X
      │     X X   │ X   X   X X X │ X           │
      │           │ X X X X │ X X X X │         X X   6
      │           │ X X X   X X │ X X X   │
      │   X       │ X X   X X │ X X       │
─────────────────────────────────────────────────────────
      │       X │ X   X X X X │           │ X X
      │         │       X X X │           │ X X
      │   X     │ X       │           │             X   7
      │         │       X     │   X X X X │
      │         │         X   │     X X   X │
─────────────────────────────────────────────────────────
X X   │         │       X X │           │ X X         X   8
─────────────────────────────────────────────────────────
      │         │ X X     │   X       X │   X
      │       X │   X   X │   X       X │   X   X
X     │         │   X     │   X         │ X X         9
X     │         │         │   X         │   X
X   X │         │         │   X         │   X
```

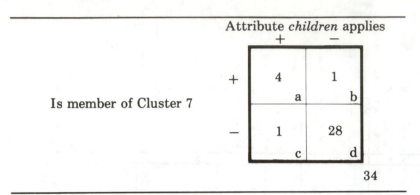

Figure 4.3. **Tabulating Attribute Criteriality**

Table 4.5. **Criteriality of Attributes Occurring in Cluster 7**

Attribute	Criteriality
Hot weather	.05
A drunk	.01
Careless	.05
Hot remedy	.01
Chills	.12
Headache	.01
Temperature	.15
Bones ache	.03
Body aches	.01
Knocks out	.05
Go to doctor	.01
Lose appetite	.04
Grave	.08
Weakening	.08
Contagious	.12
Children's illness	.64
Little, brief	.07
From a fall	.13
Vomiting	.03

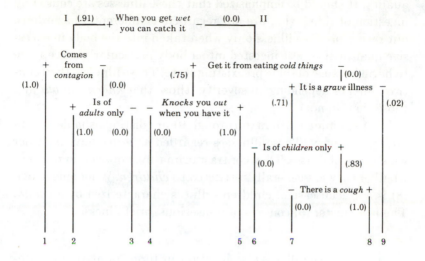

Figure 4.4. **Tree Arrangement of Highly Criterial Attributes**

Before discussing their more general meanings, it may be useful to examine Figure 4.4 in more detail.

The first attribute *(wet)* was selected as the most highly criterial of a set of highly criterial attributes that generally correspond to cluster E (Figure 4.2). It serves to sort out those illnesses that, in folk understanding, have their source in unfortunate or inadvertent contacts with environmental hazards, such as water, rain, moist ground, cold air, and fluctuating weather. These agents, primarily because of their cold qualities, impinge on bodily equilibrium and create imbalances that result in illness (see Chapter Three). These illnesses (cluster I, Figure 4.1) are then further distinguished as to whether or not they are considered a result of *contagion*[7] or are restricted to *adults*.

Those lacking the attribute *wet* and making up major cluster II are, in general, illnesses that, in contrast with those in cluster I, do not result from contact with any external hazard. Rather, they are regarded as primarily due to internally initiated conditions. These internal conditions may involve excess "cold" or "heat" or may not involve a temperature imbalance at all. Illnesses having the attribute *cold things* may result from an excess of foods having a cold quality. It should be emphasized that these illnesses are caused by ingestion of things that are not regarded as inherently hazardous, but rather produce illness only when taken into the body in excessive quantities or else ingested into a body particularly susceptible to harm because of some preexisting state. These illnesses then contrast further depending on severity (those that *knock you out* and those that do not).

The remaining clusters (6 through 9) are distinguishable first in terms of gravity. Those illnesses regarded as *grave* have a rather wide range of causes. They contrast primarily, however, in terms of whether they are generally restricted to *children*. Whooping cough (8) is a special case of children's illness characterized by a *cough*. The last cluster (9) consists of nonserious, brief illnesses.

Analysis of the illness classification in terms of attribute criteriality has yielded a set of characteristic attributes that contrast significantly between categories. We can go beyond the specifics of the model in Figure 4.4 and suggest the more general distinctions they represent. These distinctions do not derive in any strictly operational fashion from the model but rather represent a less formal, more intuitive, explanation of the findings.

First, there appears to be an overall external versus internal locus of cause distinction, in which illnesses resulting from contact with hazardous agents in the external environment contrast with those resulting from internally initiated imbalances.[8] The division between the two major clusters in Figure 4.1 reflects this distinction quite clearly, as discussed above, and is represented by the highly criterial attribute *wet*. The attribute *cold things* distinguishes those internally initiated illnesses that come about through diet-related imbalances from those involving other kinds of upsets. It is apparent on other grounds as well that this external-internal cause distinction has a general significance. One informant, asked to characterize the types of illnesses existing in Pichátaro, responded:

> There are illnesses according to the weather, that come from changes of temperature, it may be the winter. . . . There is also a class of illnesses that are personal illnesses, that are very *particular* [individual].

He went on to explain that the weather often acts to "decontrol" the body.

Pichatareños see the external environment as containing a variety of menaces to their well-being, which they must constantly recognize and deal with. Rain and moisture are particularly prominent ones. For example, we often observed people looking toward a cloud-filled sky and commenting "much illness, pure illness." When we met someone on the street in rainy weather, a common response to the greeting "What are you doing?" was "Resisting the water!"

In contrast, "personal" illnesses may come from, among other things, improper or insufficient diet, anger, fright, weakness, or lack of cleanliness.[9] Significantly, none of these causes involves the direct action of some external agent, but rather derives from the failure to maintain a healthful internal balance: this informant spoke of the *relojamiento del cuerpo,* referring to the need to regulate the body, provide proper personal care, and maintain a proper emotional state.

Thus there are two kinds of threats to a Pichatareño's well-being: he must be able to recognize and defend himself against external threats to his health; and he must continually attend to his bodily intake and emotional state to guard against upsets. His ability to identify sources of illness, however he may define them, is important, and failure to do so has, in native theory, potentially severe consequences for the accomplishment of the tasks and goals of everyday life.

A distinction between external and internal causal conditions has also been described as an important feature of folk medical beliefs in the Mayan area of southern Mesoamerica (Adams 1952; Cosminsky 1977b; Douglas 1969). In these cases, illness is often explained as the result of an interaction between the two—an internal condition (such as a heated state) that predisposes one to illness, and an external condition or agent (such as a cold rain) that precipitates the actual illness. Although Pichatareños sometimes report such interactions (see the example of Demetrio's pneumonia in Chapter Three), they more frequently attribute illness to a single causal condition. To cite an internally initiated imbalance as the cause of an illness is, in most cases, to assert the absence of any significant direct external causal agent. This is not to say that an internal imbalance could not, ultimately, be due to the presence or action of some agent external to the individual. For example, one woman explained that her case of *bilis* ('bile') was due to strong anger; this in turn was "caused" by a chance encounter with a belligerent drunk. Here, however, what was involved was not an interaction between a predisposing internal condition and a precipitating external condition. Rather it was a simple chain of causal events. In general, native theories about levels of illness causation, with each level requiring different sorts of treatment actions (see Nash 1967), do not characterize medical beliefs in Pichátaro.

Second, Pichatareños make a major distinction among illness types on the basis of seriousness. Two of the attributes in Figure 4.4 relate to seriousness (illnesses that *knock you out* and *grave* illnesses). Other findings support this interpretation. (Chapter Six will demonstrate how the gravity of an illness is one of the most crucial determinants of the strategy followed in seeking treatment.) For nonserious illnesses, Pichatareños generally use the available treatment options in order of cost—the lowest first. For grave illnesses, on the other hand, this ranking by cost is, ideally at least, replaced by an ordering of treatment alternatives based on the estimated likelihood of cure. The point emphasized by these findings is that the seriousness of an illness is a consideration that has substantial significance for treatment decisions. Evaluation of a given illness episode as serious carries with it important action imperatives (Fabrega 1974:114) and provides direction for actions aimed at coping with the illness.

Third, some illnesses are distinguished according to the life stage of the victim (Figure 4.4, clusters 2, 7, 8). While the majority of illness types considered may occur at any age, there are several for which child-specificity was the most highly criterial attribute. What significance does this distinction have? In terms of treatment, designation of a given occurrence as a kind of children's illness (measles, smallpox, whooping cough, *mollera caída,* and evil eye) carries with it important implications for the care that will be provided or sought for the victim. The first three of these, illnesses *de término* ('of a term'), must simply be left to run their course. Victims of these illnesses are cared for by being bedded down and kept from the cold air (weakened persons are particularly susceptible to "attacks" of air), but usually nothing more is given than a household remedy to "refresh" the victim and ease the illness along its course. Even though these are generally considered to be serious and potentially life-threatening illnesses, categorization of an illness episode as being of this type usually precludes resort to either medical or folk curing specialists. The following case illustrates this point:

> When Señora _____'s youngest daughter was eight days old, she got measles. At first, it was just a lot of fever, and the baby didn't eat or do anything. The Señora didn't know what to do, so she took her to [a local *practicante*]. He gave her some medicine, but it didn't help. Then when she saw that the baby was all broken out, she knew that it was measles and didn't do anything else for it. She says that the little girl was very, very sick.

The remaining two types of children's illnesses (*mollera caída* and evil eye) are amenable to treatment, but only with folk remedies. Medical specialists are said not to know about these illnesses. For example, out of thirty-three cases of *mollera caída* which were recorded, in only three instances was any alternative other than home treatment or a folk curer utilized. In the three cases when medical personnel were consulted, they are said to have been unable to cure the illness. Strategies for providing treatment for illnesses identified as a type of children's illness, will be closely constrained, then, by these special considerations.

For other illnesses, young persons, especially preverbal children and infants, are likely to receive more costly treatment and to be seen by a curing specialist earlier than adults. Children are in general thought to be less resistant to illness than adults, a belief reinforced by a relatively high infant mortality rate. The inability of infants to verbalize their symptoms also appears to engender increased concern in their relatives, which leads to earlier and more frequent use of the higher cost treatment alternatives. In these contexts, the life stage of the victim is one factor in the assessment of the seriousness of a given illness. The life stage distinction, then, is one which has a general significance in the formulation of plans for coping with illness.

Readers familiar with Mesoamerican ethnomedicine may be

struck by only a moderate mention of the "hot"-"cold" distinction in proposing an explanation for how the illness types have been found to group. This distinction is widely reported as the central feature of folk medical beliefs in Mesoamerica (Currier 1966; Foster 1953, 1967; Harwood 1971; Ingham 1970; Logan 1973), as well as a primary classificatory principle for foods, plants, animals, and other objects in the environment (Molony 1975; W. Madsen 1955). It should be clear that in Pichátaro as well these are significant concepts in beliefs about illness (see Chapter Three) and certainly many of the question frames (Table 4.2) involve this principle. However, analysis of attributes relating specifically to "hotness" and "coldness" in terms of their criteriality has shown that overall the distinction does not accurately account for cluster membership. Examination of the patterning of attributes across clusters (Table 4.4) reveals that "hot"- and "cold"-caused illnesses occur in both major clusters (I and II in Figure 4.1), indicating that this division is not primarily along "hot"-"cold" lines. Similarly, within major cluster II, the distinction between illnesses from eating cold things does not partition the illnesses as being caused by "coldness" and "hotness," since for many of the types in this cluster these qualities are either of minor importance or inapplicable. Again, this attribute distinguishes between illnesses stemming from diet-linked imbalances and those involving other sorts of internally initiated imbalances. None of the nine smaller clusters were found to be primarily characterized by one or the other of these qualities.

If the above classification does in fact relate to the kinds of distinctions that are important to Pichatareños when they must deal with illness, why has the "hot"-"cold" distinction not been more apparent? This distinction is primarily a theory of illness causation. Particular illnesses are defined in terms of the nature of the upset assumed to be involved—for example, excess "heat," excess "cold," displaced "heat." However, most people are also interested in the conditions and situations that lead up to these states of disequilibrium, so that they may avoid them, and in their consequences (in terms of discomfort, danger to life, and impaired abilities), so that they can take appropriate steps to deal with them. It is to these considerations that the classification relates. D'Andrade, in his analyses of Mexican and American illness beliefs, has made clear this disjunction between features that serve to define particular illness states, and those that are most important in accounting for how people actually categorize illness (D'Andrade 1976; D'Andrade, et al., 1972). Presumably if the present study were to be done exclusively with native curers, the resulting categories might much more consistently relate to specific etiologies. In the United States, for example, the ways in which physicians categorize illness differ substantially from those of the population in general. The same illnesses are dealt with by different kinds of people and with different purposes, and therefore the distinctions vary.

A Pichatareño would certainly consider the "hot" or "cold" quality of an illness in choosing what remedy to administer during home treatment. However, the more general decision as to whether or not to attempt home treatment, rather than consulting, say, a local curer or a physician, would depend more upon considerations such as the seriousness of the illness and the life stage of its victim.

Thus, the distinctions that best explain the illness categories existing in the data are also among the more important considerations involved in actions aimed at preventing and alleviating illness. Classifications based primarily on etiological principles (such as the "hot"-"cold" theory) do not necessarily reflect the types of knowledge most significant for purposive activities concerned with illness (contrast G. Foster 1976). The methods described here are useful, first, in determining categorical relationships inherent in illness belief data, and second, in suggesting the distinctions underlying these categories.

Earlier I pointed out that this study is concerned both with what people in Pichátaro believe to be true of illness, and with those institutional arrangements and individual decision-making processes that determine what they do about illness. The previous chapter described the basics of medical belief in the community, and this chapter has demonstrated that the structuring of illness beliefs tends to conform with how this knowledge is used in purposive action. In the following chapters we will consider the range of possible courses of action that may be taken in treating illness (Chapter Five), and how these choices are made (Chapter Six).

5

Alternatives in Treating Illness

The present set of options available to the people of Pichátaro in treating illness is the product of several traditions. Some treatment alternatives are largely indigenous—grounded in medical principles introduced by the Spanish beginning in the sixteenth century. Others represent, and are controlled by, the dominant national society, and their accessibility is determined by factors beyond the control of the local community. Still others appear to mediate between these two traditions. This chapter describes the therapeutic options largely from the perspective of the local community. We will examine the features of each alternative and their significance for treatment decisions. In the final chapter we will return to the issue of extra-community determinants of the health-care decision-making process.

As I mentioned in Chapter One, previous studies of the utilization of treatment resources in situations similar to Pichátaro's have tended to conceptualize the process as involving only two choices—folk and modern medicine. Pichatareños do in fact recognize such a contrast when they distinguish between those alternatives involving *remedios caseros* ("folk remedies," literally 'household remedies') and those involving *remedios médicos* ('medical,' or 'doctors' remedies'). It is clear, however, that there are a number of other ways in which treatment alternatives contrast, and these may often have an even greater significance in treatment decisions. Moreover, in Pichátaro people recognize more than one alternative involving modern medicine, and the considerations leading to the choice of one as compared with another are quite different. The same is also true of those alternatives involving traditional medicine. It is apparent, then, that a necessary initial step in the study

102

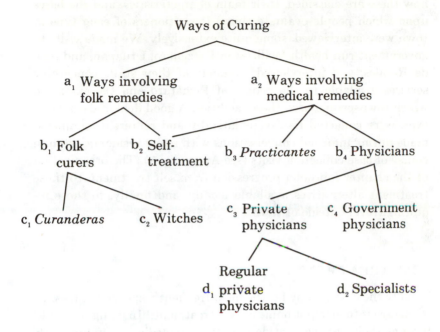

Figure 5.1. **The Pichátaro View of the Available Treatment Alternatives**

of treatment choices is an understanding of what Pichatareños view as the major available alternatives for the treatment of illness.

Figure 5.1 depicts the principal ways of curing that informants recognized and used. At the most general level is a distinction between ways of curing that involve folk remedies and those that involve modern medical remedies. Those involving folk remedies include both self-treatment and local curers of two types. Those involving modern medical remedies include physicians of several types, *practicantes,* who are local nonphysician practitioners of Western medicine, and, again, self-treatment. We shall consider each of the alternatives included in Figure 5.1.

These materials were obtained in a variety of ways. We used formal interviews to determine the perceived treatment alternatives, how these are classified, their main characteristics, and the bases upon which people evaluate them. Practitioners of each type in town were interviewed, some quite extensively. We made visits to government-run health facilities in Pátzcuaro, Uruapan, and Ario de Rosales, and interviewed members of their staffs concerning services available to the people of Pichátaro and the extent to which townspeople used these facilities. A good deal of data, however, were collected less systematically and represent comments made during informal conversations with many residents, often in course of case collection visits (see Appendix A). The organization of the chapter follows a progression from self-treatment, to those treatment alternatives available locally, and finally, to those requiring travel outside of town.

SELF-TREATMENT

Usually the first, and by far the most frequent response to illness in Pichátaro is to attempt home or self-treatment.[1] In doing so people have at their disposal a wide variety of remedies, including both traditional herbal remedies and commercially produced types, as well as a considerable store of knowledge concerning their use. Self-treatment may thus involve either *remedios caseros* or *remedios médicos.*

Many herbal and other plant-derived remedies are known and used in Pichátaro. Informants, when questioned about them, often in just a few minutes could list twenty or thirty different remedies and the illnesses for which they are used. Women, especially, have detailed knowledge in this area. The effect of folk remedies is frequently explained in terms of their "hot" or "cold" quality (see Chapter Three), which acts to correct a bodily imbalance. Other qualities, such as bitterness or repugnance, are also recognized and said to be essential in the treatment of certain illnesses. Often, however, there is apparently no specific theory of how a given remedy acts to cure a specific illness, other than the fact that it has been considered effective in the past. One man explained:

> We know so much about *caseros* because in the past there were no
> doctors or pills here. The people couldn't go to doctors then because
> they didn't know how to speak Spanish. So our ancestors made ex-
> periments, and found out which plants and herbs worked for what
> illnesses. Now we know them because of their experiments.

In many cases, then, there is no elaborate calculation of the specific
relationship between the illness state and the quality of the remedy
(such as a "hot"-caused illness, therefore a "cool" remedy), but
rather an empirically based matching of particular herbs and illnesses that is both learned as part of the cultural tradition and acquired through personal experience.

Herbs may be prepared either for ingestion or for external application. To take internally, one boils the appropriate ingredients in
water for a length of time, and then drinks the infusion. For external use, one prepares the herbal materials similarly and then rubs
the liquid on, or else applies the herbs themselves to the appropriate part of the body.

Most medicinal plant materials are gathered in town or in the
surrounding fields and forests. Some types, such as *manzanilla*
('chamomile'), used for stomach upsets, are commonly cultivated
on houselots. There are a few women who keep on hand a variety of
herbs for sale, usually in conjunction with a street-corner vegetable
stand. Unusual local herbs, herbs not native to the area, and other
kinds of medicinal materials such as certain tree barks, are available from vendors in the Pátzcuaro market. In some instances people make special trips to towns in neighboring valleys to obtain particular medicinal plants known to grow there.

In addition to herbs, other substances are sometimes used as
remedies. The following list, from case records, gives an idea of the
variety: alcohol with salt (for colds and hangovers), one's own saliva (for risen heat), urine (for sharp stomach pains), toasted opos-
sum (also for stomach pains), salt (for colds), tomatoes (for swollen
glands in the throat), a red cloth (for heart illness), burro's milk (for
whooping cough—best if from a black burro), skunk liver (for pneumonia), bread dough (applied to the cheek for toothache), a copper

coin (for headache), pig feces (for blocked digestion), and onions (also for headache). This is only a partial list, but is perhaps sufficient to make the point that for Pichatareños the range of materials potentially useful in curing is wide indeed.

Other methods used in home illness treatment do not involve the application or ingestion of medicinal substances. A common treatment for *mal de ojo* ('evil eye'), for example, is to "clean" the victim by brushing his or her body with old, dirty clothing. This is said to remove the "irritation" causing the illness. *Mollera caída* ("caused" by a dislodging of the top of the skull—see Chapter Three) is treated mechanically either by pressing on the roof of the mouth in an attempt to rise the displaced section or by sucking on the depressed area of the scalp.

Apart from traditional folk remedies used in home treatment, Pichatareños also use a number of commercially produced remedies sold in local stores. I inventoried the medicine stocks of two stores; one had available twenty-four different remedies, the other twenty. These included aspirin tablets of various types, rubs, capsules, powders, salves and other patent medicines, as well as prescription-type drugs (widely sold over the counter) like Terramycin and Enterovioform. These remedies ranged in price from fifty centavos to about three pesos. Most households seem to have favorite brands of remedies, and relatives and friends often recommend a particular tablet or pill. These remedies are usually classified as *remedios médicos* ('medical' or 'doctor's remedies'), but are regarded as having considerably less "strength" than the types of *remedios médicos* employed by *practicantes* (lay practitioners of modern medicine) and especially by physicians. Commercial remedies are generally thought to cure through the same processes as herbal remedies, for example, because of their "hotness" or "coldness," or more broadly, in terms of the strength that they contain to counteract the strength of the illness. Therefore the use of, say, aspirin for a cold instead of a traditional remedy usually indicates no reorientation of the user's beliefs concerning how the illness occurs or its effects on the body. The increasing use of patent medicines in recent years, then, is consistent with the pragmatic, empirical attitude Pichatareños have toward illness treatment. In fact, people some-times refer to their treatment attempts specifically as "experi-ments," as in the explanation I have quoted.

Most townspeople are quite interested in illness and in learning about new ways to treat it. In attempting self-treatment it is com-mon practice to seek out the advice and suggestions of relatives and neighbors. Some people also have small "medical" guides—usually oriented toward herbal curing—to which they refer. A copy of Werner's (1975) book *Donde no hay doctor* (a medical and first-aid guide for rural Latin Americans), which we circulated during the return trip in 1977, sparked considerable interest and several re-quests for copies.

Self-treatment involves more than just the preparation and ad-ministration of an appropriate remedy. Considerable effort also goes toward protecting the victim during the period of general weakness brought about by the illness. For example, with illnesses involving a fever, the victim, especially if a child, is carefully bundled in blankets to protect him or her from harmful "attacks" of cold air, to which he or she is thought particularly susceptible. In less severe cases, the head alone may be covered with a cloth or cap. Some illnesses call for the avoidance of certain foods, so as to not add to the "hot" or "cold" imbalance. Other family members may also observe certain restrictions. We observed one case in which a woman, upon arriving at her home after a trip to Pátzcuaro, stopped for a few minutes to "cool off" before entering the room in which her sick husband lay. She explained that to come near while she was still warm from the exertion of the trip would have en-dangered him. In another case, a woman scolded her younger sister for coming to see her sick infant so soon after the sister had re-turned from a visit to the cemetery. In serious cases of measles in children, the father is expected to suspend normal work activities outside of the home and to stay close to the child. His absence at such a time is said to greatly endanger the child.

Thus, an occurrence of illness is of concern to the whole house-hold, and most of its members are in some way involved in its treat-ment. There are, however, recognized limitations on what may be accomplished through home treatment, and it sometimes becomes apparent that a specialist's knowledge and remedies are required. In these cases a number of courses of action may be followed.

FOLK PRACTITIONERS

Curers

Curanderas ('curers') are persons skilled in the use of folk remedies in treating illness, who provide their services for a fee to others. There are at least fifteen such folk-curing specialists in Pichátaro, although the exact number is difficult to determine since there is no formal recruitment to the curing role, and individuals vary greatly in the extent of their involvement. While the term *curandera* may readily be applied to these specialists, more often they are simply referred to as "those who know how to cure." Curers in Pichátaro are almost exclusively women, and are usually middle aged or older, illiterate, and natives of Pichátaro. Some curers are also midwives, although this is not generally the case. We interviewed ten curers, including three with whom we maintained continuing, in-depth discussions.

The majority had mothers (and often grandmothers) who were curers, and said that they learned how to cure from them. One who did not explained that her abilities grew out of the necessity of treating the illnesses of her own numerous children; gradually her skills had become known and sought by other relatives and ulti- mately by townspeople in general. Another claims to have learned to cure from a book that was read to her. Several attributed their curing talents to God, or said that they "cure with God's help."

For almost all curing is not a full-time, nor particularly profitable, occupation. Only two appeared to derive their living mainly from curing. One explained that "you just don't earn much with this." Curers uniformly complain of frequent nonpayment for their services, and feel that people pay them much less than what their efforts merit. The average payment for a cure, which may in- volve several visits, is around fifteen pesos.

Curers use folk herbal remedies almost exclusively. Occasionally they use ointments purchased in pharmacies in Pátzcuaro, but pills, capsules, and injections are not part of their treatments. They consider herbal remedies as "natural," befitting "natural" [2] people, and more effective and safer than doctors' remedies. Most curers have their own special remedies, whose herbal ingredients they do not reveal to the client. Many of the materials used are gathered on the lands around Pichátaro, and those not native to the area are usually purchased from herb dealers in Pátzcuaro.

Most curers will treat a variety of illness types, although there is de facto specialization since people tend to bring them some illness types more frequently than others. In particular, curers tend to get disproportionately greater numbers of cases involving gastrointestinal disorders and emotion-based illnesses (in the local view of illness causation), and fewer numbers of cold and flu-like illnesses. Curers also treat children and infants more frequently than adults. *Curanderas* do not usually treat illnesses attributed to witchcraft, although two admitted that they had on occasion. Witchcraft problems are generally taken to another kind of folk practitioner.

Two curers in Pichátaro are specialized. One treats mainly burns, using a special remedy of her own manufacture. The other, the sole male curer of this type in Pichátaro, specializes in the treatment of evil eye and sprained and twisted joints. He was never referred to as a *curandero,* but simply as one good at curing these types of illnesses.[3]

Curers' reputations depend mainly upon the length of time they have been active, and their overall record in successfully treating the illnesses brought to them. Instances in which they have "cured" people after unsuccessful treatment by a physician are particularly significant; such cases are often recounted by people who wish to emphasize the skills of a particular curer. Whatever the actual therapeutic effectiveness of the treatments provided by curers, it is clear that they both consider themselves, and are widely considered by townspeople, to be sincere, honest, and often effective ministers to the sick.

The following excerpts from field notes, describing a particular case and the circumstances surrounding it, illustrate some general features of the curer's practice in Pichátaro.

Francisco G. mentioned that his eight-year-old daughter Lupe had not been well for the past few weeks. She has little appetite, looks thin, and doesn't want to play very much. She apparently has had mild diarrhea for a while, but she has been fairly active.

Yesterday afternoon we visited the G_____'s again and Francisco mentioned that they had decided to "do something" about Lupe's condition. Up until now they had been giving her some pills from Elias's store, but they didn't seem to be doing any good. That evening they were going to take her to Francisco's *compadre* Rafael [a *practicante* who uses Western medical remedies] to see if he had a medicine that would help her. After the visit to Rafael they would stop by and see us.

When they arrived we were told that they had just come from Francisco's Aunt Juana, a well-known local *curandera*. I asked why they had not taken Lupe to Rafael as they had planned. Francisco said that he had talked to his mother about the illness, and she related a case that she had heard about. A woman had been troubled by diarrhea for months and had gone to several doctors, all to no avail. Finally she went to Doña Juana and was cured. This case apparently convinced Francisco that he should take Lupe to Juana rather than to Rafael.

At the first visit, from which they had just returned, Juana applied an herbal remedy to Lupe's abdomen and told them to bring her again the following morning. Francisco invited me to come along.

We arrived at Juana's house at about eleven A.M. We seated ourselves around the small hearth in the center of the room, while Lupe sat next to Juana on the bed. She began to rub a remedy (water in which various herbs had been boiled) on Lupe's stomach and back. Lupe giggled some as the treatment continued. Juana commented that the child's stomach seemed "less tight" than it had the night before when she had given the first treatment. Lupe lay on the bed with her dress raised, exposing her stomach. Juana kept a shawl over the girl as she worked. . . . This was the extent of the actual treatment, which took about five minutes.

Juana had explained that the illness was *empacho* ('blocked digestion'), and that its cure required three treatments. She emphasized that after the third visit, to be made that afternoon, the child would be cured. . . .

The remainder of our visit—another half hour or so—was mainly spent chatting about Francisco's family. Juana's knowledge of his relatives was encyclopedic, even though the kinship connection by which he calls her "aunt" is quite distant. Juana also described other cases that she had cured, many of them, she said, after the doctors had been unable to help. Her daughter-in-law dropped in for a few minutes, and told of how Juana has taken care of all her children's illnesses, and that not one of the ten has died. . . .

As we left, Francisco gave Juana five pesos and said that he would give her more later. We also took with us a cup of the remedy, which Lupe was to drink later mixed with bicarbonate of soda. Asked what was in the remedy, Francisco said that he didn't know—"only Juana knows"—but he guessed that it had several herbs in it, all cooked together.

In further conversation after the session with Juana, Francisco explained that he has more faith in folk remedies. He said that doctors can often harm you, by giving you too much medicine or the wrong kind. He also mentioned that doctors are expensive, and if one doesn't have a lot of money they can't be consulted.

Curers are not primarily known for their diagnostic skills but rather for their knowledge of an appropriate remedy for the problem presented to them. Treatment proceeds in a relaxed and friendly atmosphere, as the above case shows, with clear assurance that the patient's condition is improving and that he or she will soon be well. Curers' services are readily available and convenient. The costs involved are low even by local standards, and payment may be delayed if money is not available at the time of treatment.

An important attribute of the different classes of practitioners is the extent to which their knowledge about illness varies from that of Pichatareños in general. This feature is likely to be significant in decisions to use a given class of practitioner, and also has implications for understanding the basis upon which practitioners validate their curing role. It is perhaps with the *curanderas* that this sort of variance is least clear cut and obvious. When treating illness, curers explain in folk terms easily understood by the client and provide remedies having qualities appropriate to traditional beliefs. However, such a congruence of expectations does not necessarily mean that both parties share exactly the same system of medical belief, and indeed some variation is inevitable (see Wallace 1970). The results of a study (presented in detail in Young 1979a) that investigated the nature of variation in folk medical beliefs between curers and lay persons provides some relevant findings.

The study was based on the responses of twenty Pichátaro women to a structured 396-item interview concerning their beliefs about illness. Ten of them had been previously identified as active folk curers, and ten were known not to engage in curing beyond routine home treatment within their immediate households. I compared the informants' responses to the questions (phrased to permit simple "yes"-"no" answers) and computed a measure of response similarity for each pair of individuals. I then used multidimensional scaling to arrive at a spatial representation of the pattern of interinformant agreement. This analysis showed the curers to have a pattern of close agreement. The noncurers proved much more divergent in their responses, showing no tendency to greater agreement among themselves than with the curers. The exceptions were the middle-aged and older noncurers, who tended to approximate the response pattern of the curers.

The results of the study show that, rather than two variant systems of traditional medical belief in the community, a lay and a specialized, there exists a single system of beliefs common to both lay and curer, with individuals varying according to their relative agreement with this standard. Rather than validating their curing function by commanding a specialized, esoteric body of knowledge about illness and its manifestations, the curer's practice in Pichátaro appears to depend upon specific skills in the implementation of a generally shared body of knowledge. Agreement with specific beliefs appears related to the opportunity to learn this aspect of the cultural tradition. Curers, with their family backgrounds and extensive day-to-day dealings with illness, have generally achieved a more highly patterned and consistent set of beliefs than noncurers. But since these beliefs are not exclusive to curers, greater agreement between the two may be expected as the age of the noncurers increases, as indeed the results show.

These findings are consistent with a view expressed by informants on several occasions that curers are thought successful not because they have access to knowledge about illness and its cure that is unavailable to ordinary people, but rather that they have a special skill in treatment. One man explained this in terms of "having the hand." He said that two people can make the identical remedy, but if one doesn't "have the hand," the cure won't work, while if the other "has the hand," the cure will prove effective.

Because of this tendency for curers' and noncurers' medical knowledge to dovetail, some people in the latter category, while expressing a strong commitment to traditional curing methods, infrequently consult local folk curers. This results from a feeling that, in their personal experiences with illness and successful past attempts at curing within their own households, if their remedies can't cure the illness, the curer's are equally unlikely to. Therefore, when home treatment is unsuccessful in such households, it is more likely that these people will select some treatment alternative other than a traditional curer. For this reason, a decision not to use curers does not necessarily imply a rejection of traditional methods of treating illness or of traditional beliefs about illness.[4]

Witches

Apart from the type of folk practitioners just discussed are those who specialize in witchcraft-related illnesses. Specifically of interest are three Pichátaro "specialists" whom people consult for the cure of illnesses thought to have been brought about by witchcraft ("good" witches). In contrast are others whose services may be engaged when one wishes to cause illness or other misfortune ("bad" witches). A given witch (*brujo,* or *hechicero*) usually does one or the other, but occasionally may do both.

The best known good witch in Pichátaro is a middle-aged man (Alfredo) who derives nearly his entire living from his curing activities. He is a native of Pichátaro, but spent many years away from the region working in several large Mexican cities. He says that on a number of occasions during these years he became involved with "people who knew a lot of magic" and herbal medicine sellers, and from these experiences he acquired a knowledge of curing. He now resides permanently in Pichátaro with two young daughters. A good part, but not all, of Alfredo's clientele comes from outside of town. His aid may be sought for a wide variety of purposes—such as solving marriage problems and locating lost possessions, in addition to illness treatment—giving his practice a shamanistic flavor. Superficially the treatments he administers are similar to those given by *curanderas,* since they involve herbal remedies and "cleanings" *(limpias)*—brushings with bundles of leaves and other objects. There are in fact substantial differences, however, since Alfredo introduces a very heavy magico-religious component into the treatment process, which is almost entirely absent in the treatments that *curanderas* give. He provides prayer and chanting as the remedies are applied, the room is filled with the smoke of burning incense, and several saints and other religious accoutrements are prominently displayed.

In contrast with Alfredo, who was very open and enthusiastically explained his work to me, the other two known witchcraft practitioners in Pichátaro were uncooperative and generally evasive. Alfredo claims to have taught both of them, and now complains that they have become too involved in making money and charge too much for their help. One of the two is an older woman whose curing work is only occasional. The other is a man who lives with a younger brother and his elderly mother. He is absent from town a good deal of the time and is said to do a lot of curing in Zamora. He recently built a large, and by local standards quite luxurious, house and has apparently become relatively prosperous in his work.

People are generally skeptical about these practitioners and their motives. Some accused them of being deceitful and "too lazy to do real work." Nevertheless witchcraft is real to many, if not most, Pichatareños, and almost all families with whom we became well acquainted eventually related past instances of witchcraft-caused illnesses and subsequent resort to such specialists. The overall frequency of such cases in Pichátaro, however, is difficult to determine because of the considerable sensitivity and ambivalence surrounding the subject. No doubt many illnesses in which witchcraft was suspected were not reported as such. Typically, instances in which witchcraft is believed involved are referred to obliquely, such as: "Some people said that maybe it was the *mala enfermedad,* but I don't know about that."

The amount of money charged by curers of witchcraft is quite high, regularly exceeding a thousand pesos. Undoubtedly, most people find such an illness a considerable and lasting financial setback. This expense usually comes at a time when much had already been spent on earlier, unsuccessful treatments.

Illnesses attributed to witchcraft are sometimes treated by specialists in Cherán, about an hour away from Pichátaro by bus. Cherán has a reputation as a center of witchcraft practice,[5] and particularly troublesome or severe cases may be taken there if one can afford it. Also, bands of gypsies (*húngaros,* literally 'Hungarians') occasionally pass through town offering a variety of "services," including fortune-telling and witchcraft. Townspeople are quite suspicious of gypsies, as we were able to observe on two occasions, but in at least a few cases they consulted gypsies for witchcraft-related illnesses.

Midwives

Although pregnancy and childbirth are often referred to euphemistically in Pichátaro as *enfermedad,* they are considered quite distinct from illness. Nevertheless, midwifery is a significant area of folk medical practice in Pichátaro, and some details may be of interest here.

While some *curanderas* are also *parteras* ('midwives'), this is not generally the case. There are seven or eight midwives who regularly attend births in Pichátaro. Like the curers, most learned their skills from mothers or other female relatives who were also midwives.

Midwives do much more than just attend the actual birth. Visits to the future mother may begin weeks before the anticipated delivery. During these visits the midwife gives massages and advises on diet and activities. Following the delivery, she visits daily for a week or two, continuing the massages and making sure that the new mother "gets well from the birth." The midwife usually takes responsibility for treating any illnesses of the mother or child during this period. It is here that there is some overlap in the midwife and curer roles.

The main consideration upon which a given midwife's reputation depends is whether or not women and infants under her care have died. A mother's death is particularly damaging in this regard. Two of the most respected and experienced midwives in town both reported that no woman they have attended has ever died. Another, however, who reportedly attended many births in past years, has seen a drastic reduction in her practice since such a death occurred.

One of the younger and most active midwives in Pichátaro has begun to acquire a degree of official certification for her work. Through the local Cultural Mission she was asked to participate in a one-month course being given at CREFAL,[6] designed to teach traditional midwives modern obstetrical practices. It is not clear, however, to what extent newly learned methods have been incorporated into her work. She explained that often what the doctors taught in the course contradicted her own understanding. She never openly disagreed with them, however, but just resolved to continue as she always had before. She is the only folk practitioner in Pichátaro who has made an attempt to acquire any sort of modern medical sanction.

We were able to get data on 256 Pichátaro births, most of which occurred over the past twenty years. They were obtained from the same sample of sixty-two households from which the illness case histories were collected. Of these births, over 96% were attended by midwives, and only 4% by physicians. Clearly childbirth is one area of health care almost completely dominated by traditional rather than modern medical practitioners. The reasons for this almost universal preference for midwives over physicians appear to be cost, convenience, and perceived quality and duration of care. The average fee charged by a midwife is around a hundred pesos, whereas a hospital delivery in Pátzcuaro attended by a doctor costs a thousand pesos or more. Delivery at home is also much more convenient and provides a familiar atmosphere in which traditional practices relating to postpartum diet and activity restrictions may be observed. As I pointed out earlier, midwives attend to the mother for extended periods both before and after the birth, and provide considerable reassurance and advice. With a physician-attended delivery, however, no such relationship exists. Contacts are brief, and the period during which care is provided is much shorter.

Of those births occurring over the five years preceding this study, which generally corresponds to the period of increased accessibility to Western medical treatment in Pátzcuaro, 88% were attended by a midwife, and 12% by a physician. This reflects some increase in recent years in the number of doctor-attended births, but still a heavy preference for midwives. In a number of cases the expectant mother went to a physician in advance of the birth for an examination of her general condition and to get an idea of whether or not a difficult delivery might be expected. The actual births in these cases, however, took place at the mothers' homes in Pichátaro and were attended by traditional midwives. In most cases of doctor-attended births there had been an early indication of a difficult birth. It is hard to say with certainty, then, whether the somewhat increased proportion of physician-attended births in recent years represents a growing trend, or rather a more stable pattern in which normal deliveries will continue to be attended by midwives, and potentially difficult ones taken to doctors. In any event, it is likely that traditional midwifery will continue to be an important aspect of folk medical practice in Pichátaro for some time to come.

LOCAL WESTERN MEDICAL RESOURCES

Although no physicians regularly practice in Pichátaro, there are nevertheless several local sources of "scientific" medical treatment. The main ones are: 1. a lay doctor; 2. a small dispensary operated by the local Catholic nuns; and 3. the nurse-staffed National Indian Institute (I.N.I.) medical post. The principal distinction between the curers described in the previous section and these is, of course, that the former use folk remedies in their treatments while the latter use modern medical remedies. Those in the present class of curing specialists are usually referred to in Pichátaro as *practicantes* ('practitioners').[7] All three *practicantes* claim to have received some medical training and usually charge a fee for their treatments. The average cost of a visit to a *practicante* is around seventeen pesos, only slightly more than the average cost of a curer's treatment.

The most frequently utilized *practicante* at the time of the study was also the only male (Rafael). He is a middle-aged native of

Pichátaro who has provided medical treatment for a number of years. Rafael has an above-average education (nine years of schooling), but his only training in Western medicine was a year he spent working as an assistant to a rural doctor. He describes this experience as a "course in nursing." He also owns a number of medical texts and first-aid guides, clearly displayed in his home, which he sometimes refers to when people come for care. Before the construction of the road connecting Pichátaro to the Pátzcuaro-Uruapan Highway in the early 1970's, Rafael's practice was more extensive than at present. However, he still provides a relatively high proportion of the treatments involving Western medical remedies in Pichátaro. Only a portion of his livelihood derives from his curing work.

Rafael is frequently consulted in cases of *gripa* and other cold-like illnesses, for which he almost invariably gives an injection. He keeps on hand a variety of prescription-type drugs (which he apparently purchases by mail) as well as at least one special tonic of his own manufacture. Occasionally when he does not have a given drug on hand he writes out its name (a "prescription") and sends the person to a pharmacy in Pátzcuaro to buy it.

He attributes his popularity to the fact that he is a native of the town and understands Tarascan. He says that older people especially prefer going to him rather than a doctor in Pátzcuaro because they can make themselves more easily understood using Tarascan. Opinion on Rafael's skills varies. Some people feel that he is the equal of a physician, and even refer to him as "*el doctor* Rafael." Most, however, feel that he possesses more limited knowledge and skills. Rafael seems to have unusually extensive *compadrazgo* ties in all parts of town, and it is likely that his popularity as a *compadre* choice is due in large part to the valued aid he can provide.

The same general type of treatment available from Rafael may also be obtained from the local Catholic nuns, who maintain a small dispensary in the convent adjacent to the church. One of the three nuns has had a correspondence school course in nursing, and all seem to have had some instruction in basic first aid and hygiene as part of their training. They are less willing than Rafael to treat illnesses that appear serious, and report that they often advise patients to go to a doctor in such cases. While no records are kept, it appears that children much more frequently than adults are taken to the nuns. Fees are charged only to cover the cost of the medication, and at times there is no charge at all if the person says he or she cannot afford it. The nuns consider their medical work as one of the social services they provide to the community. None of the three is a native of the area or knows Tarascan. The nuns are away from town fairly often—and absent throughout June, July, and August for vacations—so their services are rather frequently unavailable.

Another local source of Western-style therapy, and the only one having any significant degree of official sanction and support, is the I.N.I. medical post. This facility is located in one room of the town hall, facing the main plaza. It contains an examination table (made of planks and sawhorses), a few chairs, tables, limited examination equipment, and a shelf holding a fairly large assortment of medications. Its scheduled hours are nine to two o'clock, and then four until six. However, it was often observed to open late and not at all in the afternoon hours. "Weekends" were occasionally expanded to include both Friday and Monday. The sole nurse who staffs the medical post was trained in a one-year practical nursing course at the I.N.I. Coordinating Center in San Cristóbal de las Casas, Chiapas. She was in her early twenties at the time of the study, and is a native of a town on Lake Pátzcuaro. She is also on vacation during the summer months.

The I.N.I. post is the only treatment alternative in Pichátaro which keeps records of patient visits. They show that around half of all cases involved *gripa* ('cold,' 'flu'), with lesser numbers of cases of anemia, diarrhea, wounds, coughs, and sore throats (these are all the nurse's designations). While such complete data are lacking for the other two *practicantes* (the nuns and Rafael), there is apparently no great difference in the types of illnesses treated by all three. However, the age and sex distribution for the medical post (Figure 5.2) suggests one probable difference. It shows that males are treated here much less frequently than females.[8] Since children are almost always brought by their mothers, only about an eighth of all patient visits are by males old enough presumably to have

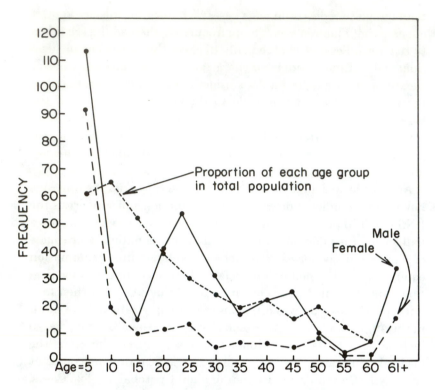

Figure 5.2. **Age and Sex Distribution of I.N.I. Medical Post Patients**

come on their own. One informant explained that "the men go to
the man, and the women to the woman," and indeed this does seem
to be the case. Men are apparently reticent to seek the advice of a
young woman, preferring to go to the nuns or, especially, to Rafael.
The nurse's most frequent patients, apart from the children, are
other women of approximately her own age.

It is inaccurate to assume that *practicantes* operate totally apart
from the local system of folk medical beliefs and practices. Although they use scientific medical remedies almost exclusively,
nevertheless, in varying degrees, they incorporate folk concepts
into their treatment practices and explanations of illness. Several
cases were recorded in which a parent took a child to a *practicante*,
only to be told that the illness was really *mollera caída* ('fallen fon-

tanel') or *mal de ojo* ('evil eye'), and could only be successfully treated by a curer using folk remedies. Rafael frequently explained *gripa* in terms of contact with "cold" and "airs." The *practicante* role is thus able to incorporate scientific medical remedies, which in many cases are considered faster acting than herbal remedies, without necessarily contradicting local conceptions of illness causation and process.

In addition to *practicantes,* there are other types of personnel who have occasionally provided Western-style medical treatment in Pichátaro, or who perform an auxiliary function in such treatment. Periodic visits of doctors have been arranged sporadically over a number of years. Soon after the road was put in, the town priest persuaded a physician friend to begin weekly visits. Apparently few people consulted him, and his visits were reported to have ended rather quickly. In 1972–1973 a physician practiced for a year in Pichátaro. He was a *pasante,* or recent medical school graduate, fulfilling the social service obligation of all new physicians (and other professionals) in Mexico. He held consultations in the same facility more recently occupied by the I.N.I. nurse. The physician, however, was under the auspices of the *Secretaría de Salubridad y Asistencia* (the Ministry of Health and Public Assistance, abbreviated S.S.A.), and the post was designated as a C-class Health Center (the most modest class of health center regularly staffed by a physician). The amounts of money officially charged at this center were fairly low, involving a consultation fee of a few pesos and a discounted price for the medication.

However, the facility does not appear to have been very extensively used. Few people reported having consulted with the doctor themselves, although they said that he was "sometimes" used by people they knew. Generally *pasantes* are considered inexperienced beginners, and apparently there was no exception in this case. Also, a few people hinted that the *pasante* might have "padded" the charges made to patients. S.S.A. officials in Uruapan explained that failure to restaff the Health Center at the termination of this doctor's stay was caused by the increased availability of transportation to Pátzcuaro brought about by the new road. They apparently believed that Pichatareños now had somewhat easier access to the much larger A-class Pátzcuaro Health Center. Personnel were thought best assigned to more isolated towns.

During our residence in Pichátaro in 1975–1976, a physician from Morelia (the state capital) began making biweekly visits to town, holding consultations in a private home. His availability was not very widely known, however, and his services seemed at times to entail considerable delay. In one case a woman suffering from *bilis* ('bile') visited him. The doctor told her that he did not have the appropriate medication with him but would bring it on the next visit. He forgot it, however, and the remedy was ultimately delivered more than a month after the initial consultation.

Shortly before our departure in 1977, a fourth-year[9] medical student from the University of Michoacán in Morelia began spending weekends in Pichátaro in order to provide medical care. He came sponsored by the I.N.I. Coordinating Center in Pátzcuaro, which also was to provide a stock of medications. The student's expenses were to be covered by a five peso consultation fee collected from each patient treated. His presence in town had been formally approved (although with much delay) by the town authorities, and his availability announced over loudspeaker setups on the day of his arrival. At present it is not known whether these visits have continued, or what the town's reaction has been.

During 1977 a dentist from Uruapan also began making weekly visits to Pichátaro, operating out of a small room adjacent to one of the principal stores in town. This was the first time that any sort of dental care had been available locally, and it seemed well received. Unfortunately no data are available on fees or on the number of patients. The range of services was limited because of the lack of facilities.

The Cultural Mission that resided in town in 1975–1976 and in 1976–1977 (see Chapter Two) included a nurse, but her activities mainly involved teaching hygiene classes, and only incidentally treating illness. The medications available to her were quite limited.

There are also a number of young women in Pichátaro who have hypodermic syringes and know how to use them. Many learned this skill from either the present or previous Cultural Mission nurses.

These women are not practitioners, for they neither prescribe medication nor take responsibility for the care of sick people. Rather, they simply provide their service, for a small fee, when the medication has been previously obtained (from a *practicante,* pharmacy, or doctor) and must be injected.

Examination of the recent history of Western medical practice in Pichátaro shows that the most frequently used practitioners have been those whose abilities and limitations are known to townspeople through long-term personal experience. Formal training and official sponsorship do not necessarily result in extensive use unless accompanied by personal acquaintance. A practitioner must demonstrate his or her skills, and it is this successful demonstration that leads to a demand for services.

MEDICAL RESOURCES IN PATZCUARO

Apart from the above sources of local treatment, Pichatareños utilize medical treatment in the town of Pátzcuaro, located about an hour away by bus. Pátzcuaro has physicians in private practice, a government-run health center, and pharmacies.

Of these the most preferred, but generally the most costly, is treatment by a private doctor. There are five or six in Pátzcuaro who are regularly visited by people from Pichátaro; two are particularly well known. Pichatareños prefer private doctors, as opposed to government-employed ones, because they generally have a shorter wait and get a more elaborate examination. They are particularly impressed by stethoscopes, X rays, and laboratory procedures such as blood and urine analysis, which they feel allow the doctor literally to "see inside" one's body to determine what is wrong. Doctors in Pátzcuaro are thus considered to be expert diagnosticians, as well as specialists possessing powerful remedies. They are, however, expensive. The average cost of a physician's treatment is around 150 pesos (the better part of a week's wages for a day laborer). In very serious illnesses, in which several visits are required, the cost may exceed a thousand pesos. People therefore consider the cost to be unpredictable and feel that they must be prepared for the worst when they consult a doctor. The fact that they are paying for these services, however, makes most feel that they have some control over, and the doctor some concern with, the quality of the medical care.

A variety of medical services are also available at the Class A Pátzcuaro Health Center operated by the federal Ministry of Health and Public Assistance. These facilities are housed in a modern building appropriately adjacent to the Basilica of the Virgin of Health. The Center includes a general outpatient clinic as well as specialized maternity and children's clinics, services in dermatology and dentistry, and a laboratory. At the time of our study, the staff included a director, two *pasantes* or recent medical school graduates, two established Pátzcuaro doctors who worked at the Center part time, several nurses, and other administrative and auxiliary personnel. Physicians' services were usually available from around 9 A.M. until 2 P.M., five days a week. The Center collects a consultation fee of a few pesos, and charges at a discount for medications. At times, however, the Center does not have a given medication on hand, and it must be purchased at a pharmacy at full price. As a general rule, a visit to the Center costs about half what a visit to a private physician would cost for a comparable illness. Despite this, the Center is used much less frequently than private doctors (the ratio is about one to three) because people consider the treatment there to be of lower quality. Visits usually involve a long wait, and consultations are often said to be cursory, involving only a few questions and no physical examination at all. People generally believe that all of the physicians at the Center are *pasantes,* and therefore inexperienced and not "real" doctors. Sometimes they reported that they had not seen a doctor at all, but rather a nurse who had listened to their complaint, relayed it to the doctor, and then returned with the medication.[10] The fact that the doctor's salary is paid by the government makes some feel that he is disinterested in the outcome of the treatment. Thus, in terms of the standards by which Pichatareños judge modern medical treatment, the services provided at the Pátzcuaro Health Center are deficient. Perhaps the Center's chief problem is chronic underfunding—a factor well beyond the control of the staff.

Residents of Pichátaro occasionally go to pharmacies in Pátzcuaro to buy medication with no consultation other than with the pharmacist or clerk. The customer describes the symptoms to the pharmacist, shows the problem to him if possible, and asks what remedy would be "good" for it. In most instances reported, pharmacists provided a medicine, although at times they refused to provide a remedy and advised the person to go to a doctor. Pichatareños most often use pharmacies in this manner in hopes of avoiding a physician's consultation fee; they may also be used for some less serious illnesses, in which the problem is readily describable or visible. A few people seemed to think of pharmacists as a kind of doctor, despite the significant differences in their styles of "practice." [11]

Another facility recently available to Pichatareños, but as yet little used by them, is the clinic at the National Indian Institute's Coordinating Center in Pátzcuaro. The Center's staff includes a physician who, in addition to his other duties, conducts a clinic two or three days a week. The Center opened in late 1975, and the medical services became available somewhat later. The existence of this service was therefore little known in Pichátaro at the time of this study, although presumably some would have learned of it through referral by the local I.N.I. nurse.

OTHER ALTERNATIVES

Several other treatment possibilities are sometimes chosen by residents of Pichátaro, although with less frequency than those thus far described. I include them to give a more complete picture of the relatively wide range of possible treatment that may be adopted in attempting to deal with an illness.

Other Sources of Western Medical Treatment

In addition to physicians available in Pátzcuaro, Pichatareños occasionally consult doctors practicing in the larger cities of Uruapan, Morelia, and elsewhere. Some people seem to believe that the skills and knowledge of physicians are proportional to the size of the city in which they practice.[12] Accordingly, when a doctor in Pátzcuaro has been consulted with no success, the next step, re-

sources permitting, is often to consult a doctor in Morelia. In very
rare instances, wealthier Pichatareños have resorted to facilities as
far away as, for example, the National Cancer Institute in Mexico
City. Pichatareños distinguish between "regular" doctors and "specialists," and it is to the latter that they resort in unusual circumstances. Interestingly, "specialists" are thought not so much as particularly expert in a certain branch of medical practice, but rather
as doctors more highly skilled and knowledgeable *in general*.

Another facility which recently became available to residents is
the Mexican Social Security Institute's (I.M.S.S.) Rural Hospital-
Clinic in Ario de Rosales, a town located about an hour's ride south
of Pátzcuaro (and about two hours' travel time, plus waits, from
Pichátaro). The Ario Clinic is part of a new I.M.S.S. program to
extend the availability of its medical services to rural *campesinos*
who would otherwise be ineligible to receive them.[13] It is housed in
a new, modern building and offers a wide range of medical services
including surgery and hospital care. The most interesting feature is
that all services and medications are provided without charge.
Therefore, the only direct expense associated with the use of the
Clinic is the cost of transportation, which from Pichátaro amounts
to about thirty pesos per person, round trip.

The Clinic was first announced in Pichátaro in late March 1976,
when a team of twelve employees of the I.M.S.S. visited town for
two days, signing people up to receive an identification card (the
card could also be obtained upon arrival at the Clinic itself). People
were generally willing to enroll in the program, although many
commented that the Clinic was a long way away. One common initial reaction was skepticism over the claim that the services were
indeed free. We first began to hear of people going to the Clinic
shortly before our first departure in August 1976.

During the return visit in the summer of 1977, we again surveyed
the sixty-two households in the case collection sample in order to
record illnesses that had occurred in the approximately one-year
period that had elapsed. We found that better than one out of every
five physician visits during that period had been made at the Ario
Clinic. There had, then, been a generally favorable response to the
introduction of this new treatment alternative. Doubts about the

services being free had diminished as more evidence became available. Even more significant, those who had used the Clinic gave an almost uniformly positive evaluation of the treatment they had received. In this instance many of the problems cited for the Pátzcuaro Health Center had, to a degree, been overcome.

Another factor affecting use of the Ario Clinic is cost. Assuming the ill person went with one companion, the transportation costs involved are about the same as the average total cost for a visit to the Pátzcuaro Health Center (including the charges made at the Center). In many cases, then, the costs of the two alternatives would be about equal. However, an additional feature favoring the Ario Clinic is that the cost is predictable: one always knows just how much it will be. With the Pátzcuaro Center there is always the possibility of greater expense than one anticipates. Thus, a number of factors seem to favor increased use of the new clinic. (Future data on this will be useful in evaluating some of the conclusions in Chapter Seven.)

Marginal Alternatives

Residents of Pichátaro sometimes purchase remedies from medicine vendors and herbal remedy sellers in the market in Pátzcuaro,[14] and occasionally vendors pass through Pichátaro in *carros de propaganda* (loudspeaker-equipped cars or trucks). Their products are often quite exotic (such as "bee poison with coyote liver," or "shark tablets") and are promoted with elaborate "scientific" explanations of their supposed effect on the body. These people usually have a masterful knowledge of local folk medical beliefs and cast their presentations accordingly. In most cases, vendors are considered as sources of remedies used in the home treatment of illness rather than as direct providers of treatment. On at least two occasions during this study, however, medicine sellers arrived in town and announced their availability for consultations. In these cases, the seller both provided a diagnosis of the problem and recommended a course of treatment involving, of course, their remedies. At times, then, they can constitute an alternative source of treatment, although this is quite rare. Pichatareños are fairly suspicious of their claims.

Spiritual advisors and assorted "professors" in Uruapan, Zacapu, and elsewhere often advertise over radio stations received in Pichátaro, offering to help restore health and vitality. The extent to which townspeople actually seek their assistance is not known, but it is probably infrequent. The practice of spiritualism, reported in other areas of Mexico (see C. Madsen 1965; Kearney 1977), is virtually unknown in Pichátaro.

Occasionally, for particularly prolonged or serious illnesses Pichatareños may seek supernatural aid. Such requests usually take the form of a *compromiso* ('promise,' or 'vow') made with a particular saint's image, in which the petitioner promises to fulfill some obligation, such as making a pilgrimage to the saint for a certain number of years, in exchange for divine intervention in the illness. The fulfillment of such a vow may involve arduous journeys on foot. The Christ image in the church at Nuevo San Juan Parangaricutiro, south of Uruapan, is regionally famous for such requests. Even more venerated by Pichatareños is the Christ of Carácuaro, located in the hot country of southeast Michoacán, where a massive pilgrimage is made annually.

This chapter has described the basic features of the variety of treatment options available to Pichatareños. It has thus set the foundation for the model of treatment decision making, which is developed in the following chapter. In developing the model, we will deal with four basic treatment alternatives: self-treatment, folk curers, *practicantes,* and physicians. (These are the four "ways of curing" in level b of Figure 5.1.) While the model will not deal specifically with each alternative described in the present chapter (including those at levels c and d in Figure 5.1), it does essentially encompass the entire range of available alternatives by considering these four major categories.

6

The Choice of Treatment

The treatment of illness in Pichátaro involves choosing among several alternatives, each differing from the others in a number of ways. This chapter considers the process by which these choices are routinely made. We have come to the central focus of the research, and to where it departs most significantly from the majority of previous studies of health-care utilization (see Chapter One). That is, we are concerned not with correlates of the different outcomes of this decision process, but rather with modeling the process itself. We will specify the information that people consider when faced with illness treatment decisions, the principles whereby this information is used in making choices, and the relevant external constraints. Underlying much of what follows is a concern with discovering how people reduce this potentially complex cognitive task to the point at which they are actually able to make a decision.

The working assumption is that there exists a more or less set, and generally shared, natural decision-making process for the treatment of illness that we can, in fact, discover. This assumption is justified on several grounds. Illness is a recurrent human problem with which nearly everyone must deal. Because it is recurrent and because the consequences of "wrong" choices may at times be severe, people usually develop and come to rely upon specific standards for making these choices (see Quinn 1978:219–220). Because people characteristically seek others' advice and communicate with them about their decisions, the process through which they are made is likely to be accessible through direct questioning. The subsequent test of the model developed here will also serve as a test of this working assumption.

Before describing the development of the decision model, let us consider some basic features of the data it seeks to explain. These data derive from records of 323 illnesses that occurred in a sample of sixty-two Pichátaro households. We visited each household on an approximate biweekly basis over a six-month period and made detailed case histories of each illness experienced by members of the household during that period. (See Appendix A for details on the case collection procedures.) None of the informants interviewed in developing the decision model was included in the sample households; these illness records therefore constitute an independent set of data, whose primary role is to test the model.

Table 6.1 summarizes the cases according to the number of treatment alternatives used in each. The largest number of illnesses involved use of only one treatment alternative. Fewer, but still sizable, numbers of cases involved use of two or three sources, rarely four or more. Very few reported cases involved no treatment at all (although the tendency would be not to report these during the case collection visits). In most cases in which people resorted to two or more alternatives, their choices were sequential rather than concurrent. Simultaneous use of more than one treatment source did occur, but most often a given treatment was carried out until people felt it had failed. They often explained that a given treatment was just not "cutting" the illness, or that "we could see that the illness was too strong," at which point they selected some new course of action.

Since the unit of analysis here is each instance in which a particular treatment alternative was used, and since about one-third of the cases involved use of two or more alternatives, the number of choices to be accounted for exceeds the number of illness episodes. The distribution of these choices across the four major alternatives

Table 6.1. **Number of Steps in Treatment Sequence**

Number	Frequency	Percentage
No treatment	4	1.2
One alternative	199	61.6
Two alternatives	80	24.8
Three alternatives	32	9.9
Four alternatives	6	1.9
Five alternatives	2	0.6
Total	323	100.0

Table 6.2. **Distribution of Treatment Choices**

Choice	Self-treatment	Curer	Practicante	Physician	Other	
Initial	232	24	31	23	9	
Second	7	34	35	38	6	
Third	2	9	6	21	2	
Fourth	0	2	0	5	1	
Fifth	0	0	0	2	0	
Total	241	69	72	89	18	= 489
Percentage	49.3	14.1	14.7	18.2	3.7	100

(see Chapter Five) appears in Table 6.2. About half of the choices led to self- or home treatment, with the other half fairly evenly divided among curers, *practicantes,* and physicians (including the Pátzcuaro Health Center). A small number involved other sources. These data show that the initial action taken in nearly three-fourths of all cases is to administer home treatment. Informants commented frequently that self-treatment is "always" the first thing done for an illness. However, exceptional cases did occur (about 25% of the time) that did not involve home treatment.

One important task, then, is to specify the considerations determining whether people choose self-treatment initially and, if not, when they are most likely to choose each other alternative. A second task posed by these data is the explanation of subsequent choices of treatment when more than one is made in the course of a given illness—which alternatives people choose under what conditions, and their order of use. It is to these tasks that the model must answer.[1]

DISCOVERING THE DECISION CRITERIA AND PROCESS

The extent to which the considerations involved in people's decisions are accessible through direct questioning generally depends upon how frequently communication about such decisions naturally occurs.[2] In dealing with illness treatment decisions we found that these decisions are usually made with a good deal of consultation and discussion with others. Indeed, current illnesses, and the steps being taken to deal with them, form popular topics of casual conversations in Pichátaro, especially among women. A person with sickness in the family may be called to while walking down the street, interrogated in detail about the illness, and given suggestions about remedies to try, or to whom to take the sick person. Equally as often, people actively seek such advice. Within this setting most people come to have definite ideas about what circumstances call for the use of a particular alternative, and can, as will be apparent, readily talk about them when given appropriate questioning contexts.

The first step in constructing a formal model of the choice-making process was discovery of the principal decision criteria. We accomplished this by means of the contrastive questioning or "paired comparisons" techniques suggested by Gladwin (H. Gladwin n.d.). His recommendations are basically these: questions should be contrastive rather than general ("When is it that you do X rather than Y?", instead of "How do you decide what to do?"); and questions should exhaust all choice contrasts (all possible pairs of alternatives) within the area of interest. Given the results of this type of questioning, one should then be in a position systematically to specify the range of considerations leading to the selection of each of the alternatives. The extent to which choices unanticipated by the model were then observed to occur in actual cases would indicate the degree to which the model fails to provide a complete account of the choice criteria involved. As the sole procedure for the construction of a decision-making model the paired comparison method has some important limitations, which will be discussed later. I found it, however, to be an extremely useful starting point for the development of such a model.

The basic form of the questions was as follows:

If you or another person in your household were ill, when—for what reasons—would you (consult) (use) _____ instead of (consulting) (using) _____ ?

All possible contrasting pairs of alternatives were inserted in the frame. Those included were the following (see Chapter Five): 1.

self-treatment; 2. a folk curer; 3. a pharmacy (with consultation only with the clerk or pharmacist); 4. a local *practicante;* 5. the Pátzcuaro Health Center; and 6. a private-practice physician. This resulted in thirty questions (thirty-six possible pairs, minus the six pairs in which an alternative is paired with itself). Note that each pair of alternatives was presented twice (such as, ". . . home treatment rather than a curer," and later ". . . a curer rather than home treatment"). The reverse ordering, rather than being redundant, as it might at first appear, is actually a very different question which led to the mention of additional considerations. Not all informants were familiar with all alternatives, so in a few cases we eliminated some questions from the interview.

The interview was completed with fifteen persons, eight men and seven women, of varying age, occupation, and economic status. The following excerpts illustrate the types of data that resulted:

(. . . when . . . would you use a curer instead of home treatment?)

> Not everyone knows *remedios caseros,* and sometimes it's necessary to have a curer make the remedy. It's when you don't know which remedy will serve. If you know, from your experience, what the remedy is, then you just make it at home.

(. . . a private physician instead of the Pátzcuaro Health Center?)

> When the illness is grave, and you want them to attend to it rapidly, regardless of whether it costs or not. When the cost is of no importance, just as long as they attend to you. Sometimes you have to wait a long time at the Center, and with the private doctors it costs more, but they attend to you fast. You go when the illness is very advanced and you have the money for it.

(. . . a *practicante* instead of a curer?)

> Some people have more *fe* [faith, confidence] in the nurses. If you try the *caseros* which you know are good for the illness and they

don't work, you don't go to the curer to try the same thing again.
You go to the nurses to see if they can help you. They can cure *gripa*
faster. But if you have *fe* in the curer and know that she can cure the
thing, better to go there.

(. . . a private physician instead of home treatment?)

When it is very grave and you can't cure it with *caseros*. Now
when people get something, and they can't cure it at home, they go
running to the doctor because it's *más seguro* ('more certain') there.
But you have to have the money to go.

Each question directs attention to a specific contrast between
treatment alternatives. By considering all of the responses that include a given alternative, we may construct a relatively complete
description of the considerations that routinely lead to its use. The
special virtue of the pair-by-pair questioning is that it requires the
informant to consider all possible choice contrasts. One result of
this kind of exhaustiveness is that responses were often the same for
different pairs. For example, the reason for using home or self-
treatment instead of consulting a *practicante* is the same as the
reason for using home treatment instead of a private physician:
"when it's not grave and you know the remedy for it." This is not to
say that consulting *practicantes* and physicians are equivalent
courses of action, but rather that, in this case, the two alternatives
are ranked: if there is no need to consult a *practicante* because an
illness is considered easily handled at home, then certainly there is
no need to see an expensive physician. When one would consult a
practicante instead of a physician is another question.

Case histories of past illnesses and the treatment actions taken
were also collected from each of the fifteen informants participat-
ing in the paired comparisons interviews.[3] A list of some fifty illness
types was reviewed, and cases of each type that had occurred in the
informant's household were recorded. An average of around
twenty-five cases was obtained for each of the households involved.
These data were used to check the validity of statements made in
the paired comparisons interviews through discussion of actual ill-

ness episodes and the treatment alternatives used. The case histories were collected a day or two after the paired comparison interview had been completed, and the responses reviewed. During this second interview, any instances in which informants' past actions disagreed with their earlier explanation of how they made their choices could be discussed and their explanation accordingly revised or amplified.

A second purpose in collecting the case histories was to make available data on the relative frequencies with which the six treatment alternatives included in the interviews had actually been used during the period covered. On the basis of these data, I decided to reduce by two the number of alternatives included in the formal model of choice of treatment. First, the use of pharmacies as primary sources of health care was infrequent, and in such accord with the discussion of this alternative in Chapter Five, that it seemed unnecessary to include it in the model. Second, the occasions on which the Pátzcuaro Health Center was used were relatively infrequent and sufficiently similar overall to those in which physicians in private practice were used to justify, for the purpose of the formal model, grouping these two alternatives. Thus we are left at this point with the four primary illness treatment alternatives enumerated at the end of Chapter Five—self-treatment, folk curers, *practicantes,* and physicians.[4]

Findings of the Paired Comparisons Interviews

Four criteria were consistently cited in the interviews as principal considerations, particularly in the initial choice of treatment: 1. the gravity or seriousness of the illness; 2. the knowledge and experience possessed concerning the given type of illness and its appropriate remedy; 3. the *fe* ('faith,' 'confidence') one has in the effectiveness of folk treatment and remedies *(remedios caseros)* as opposed to medical treatment and remedies *(remedios médicos),* in treating the given illness;[5] and 4. the expenses associated with some alternatives and the availability of the resources to meet them. Of the four, the gravity of the illness is the most general consideration, since it is cited as relevant to choices involving all four of the treatment alternatives. (The specific contexts within which each of the other considerations is relevant, and the choices they lead to, are described in detail later in the chapter.)

Apart from these four general considerations, the responses also contain contingency considerations. These assume that a prior treatment has not been successful and suggest what would be an appropriate alternative course of action. For example, one reason for going to a curer is when "home treatment has not been able to cure it"; a physician would be consulted "when no one else has been able to do it [cure the illness]," and so on. Throughout the responses are suggestions of orderings or sequences through which different alternatives would be used in the process of seeking a cure. These orderings vary among different informants, particularly when the responses of the relatively more wealthy are compared with those of the relatively less wealthy. The data are suggestive but limited, since they do not adequately define these orderings, nor do they clearly specify the implications that unsuccessful treatments have for subsequent choices. A second interview technique was designed to provide additional data on these issues.

Orderings of the Treatment Alternatives

I employed the second technique—that of hypothetical situations—to obtain data on the order of use of treatment alternatives, and the ways in which this ordering may vary. Taking three of the four key considerations cited above—seriousness, available resources, and knowledge of an appropriate remedy—a series of hypothetical situations was devised. A situation was described and the informant asked what the probable sequence of actions would be. The fourth consideration—one's faith in folk versus medical treatment—was not specified in order to determine for what particular choices it would be cited as relevant. This interview was completed with twenty informants, including the majority of those who had participated in the paired comparison interviews.

In the hypothetical situations each consideration was posed in a limiting condition: seriousness was either very grave or minor; available resources were described as fairly abundant or scarce; and the illness had either been successfully treated before within the household or else it was unknown. There are, of course, intermediate values between these extremes, but constraints on the length of the interview required a smaller number of values for each of the three considerations. Therefore, I decided to include only the limiting values at each end of the scale, as these were the most likely to produce clear-cut orderings of the alternatives.

Since there were three considerations, each with two values, a total of eight hypothetical situations were presented. The following examples illustrate the form in which these situations were described:

Situation	*Approximate English translation of description*
1. Serious Money available Remedy known	Let's say that there is a person that has a very grave illness. This family has a fair amount of money, because they have draft animals and have just sold one. They have had this illness before in the family, and they now know the remedy that benefited the illness on that occasion. What do you think they are going to do?
2. Serious No money available Remedy known	Let's say that there is a person that has a very grave illness. In this family money is scarce—sure they're eating, but there is just not anything left over. They have had this illness before in the family and they now know of the remedy that benefited the illness on that occasion. What do you think they are going to do?
3. Nonserious Money available No remedy known	Let's say that there is a person that has a little illness—sure they're sick, but they are not going to die of it or anything like that. In this family there is some money, because they have just come back from Mexico City where they were working. They haven't had this illness before in the family, and they really don't know what it is, or what it came from, or what the remedy is—for them it is unknown. What do you think they will do?

The particular sources of funds cited in Situations 1 and 3 were used because they are realistic in terms of the local economy and would provide enough money to allow for almost any plan of action to obtain treatment.

After each reply, informants were asked what they would do if the action just taken had been ineffective. This question was repeated until they finally said that nothing more could be done. Typically a given situation would elicit four or five such steps. The following are examples of replies to Situations 1 and 2:

Situation 1. (Informant is a thirty-year-old woman)

A First they will use the remedy that they already know will cure it.

Q What if this time the remedy doesn't help, and the illness stays the same?

A Then they will go to a doctor. If they carry a lot of money, they are going to go first to the doctor. It's more sure and quicker there.

Q What if the doctor is not able to help it either?

A They will go to another doctor who knows more, maybe in Morelia.

Q Let's say that they go to this doctor, but they still are sick?

A Now they will go to a *curandera* to see if she can cure it. Often people have more *fe* in the doctor than in the curer, but if the doctors can't cure it, they will see if the curer can because she is often able to.

Q And if the curer can't?

A Now they are going to think that it is the *mala enfermedad* [caused by witchcraft] and they'll go to Cherán, where there are good curers of witchcraft. They'll come and assure them that they will be cured, and they will find the thing that caused the illness and the person will begin to feel that he is going to get well.

Situation 2. (Informant is a forty-five-year-old woman)

A First they are going to give him the remedy that they already know of.

Q And if the illness continues the same?

A Then they will go to the nurse in the plaza or to a *curandera,* depending on what the illness is. If it's a fever or a cough or something like that you go to the nurse, but if it's a sprain or body aches or *la bilis* you go to a *curandera.*

Q Let's say that they do this, but still the illness continues. Now what will they do?

A They will have to get the money to go to a doctor. They will try to get it by borrowing, or selling some animal, or by pawning a piece of land. This is the last thing they will do, for lack of money. If they can't get quite as much they might go to the Centro de Salud [Pátzcuaro Health Center].

Q And what if even the doctor can't cure the illness?

A If it can't be cured with the doctor or with *remedios caseros,* then there's no way, and they come back sad.

The first example illustrates one of the two general orderings of choices that were evident in the data. In this ordering, the most important concern is to determine the alternative that seems most likely to cure the illness, regardless of the cost, and resort to it first. In the second ordering, however—illustrated in Situation 2—the most important consideration becomes the cost associated with each alternative, and only when these are approximately equal (as with the nurse and the curer) does consideration of the likelihood of cure become primary. The strategy in this case is to turn to the most expensive alternative, usually the physician, only as a last resort after the other less costly options have been exhausted. In fact, half of the informants thought that both a curer and a *practicante* would be consulted before a physician. The problem here, then, is to determine which situation regularly led to one, or the other, of these two orderings.

My approach was to calculate a figure expressing the percentage of agreement in the responses for each pair of hypothetical situations in the interview. These figures are given in Table 6.3.[6] They indicate several sets of situations in which informants agreed substantially on the likely sequence of treatment choices. Specifically, the responses for Situations 1 and 2 are very similar to each other when initial differences are controlled for, but are not consistently similar to any others.[7] Situations 3, 4, and 5 also show high levels of agreement, as do 6 and 7. Both 1 and 2 are associated with trying the most certain cure, regardless of cost (probability-of-cure ordered pattern), which is consistent with the fact that both situations involve serious illnesses in relatively wealthy households. Especially interesting is the similarity of Situations 3, 4, and 5. Sit-

Table 6.3. **Similarity Figures for Hypothetical Situation Responses**

		1	2	3	4	5	6	7	8
$+S^a$ $+M^b$ $+K^c$	1	1.0							
$+S$ $+M$ $-K$	2	.26	1.0						
		(.78)		1.0					
$+S$ $-M$ $+K$	3	.26	$-.29$						
$-S$ $+M$ $+K$	4	.30	$-.21$	.68	1.0				
$-S$ $-M$ $+K$	5	.05	$-.40$	.66	.66	1.0			
$+S$ $-M$ $-K$	6	$-.14$	.07	.18	.05	$-.04$	1.0		
				(.42)					
$-S$ $+M$ $-K$	7	.08	.20	.12	.12	$-.15$	.61	1.0	
					(.63)				
$-S$ $-M$ $-K$	8	$-.43$	$-.27$	.07	.07	.12	.39	.30	1.0
						(.21)			

a Seriousness: $+S$ = very grave; $-S$ = little.
b Available Resources: $+M$ = adequate; $-M$ = scarce.
c Knowledge of Remedy: $+K$ = remedy known; $-K$ = remedy unknown.

uation 3 involves a serious illness in a poor household; 4, a nonserious illness in a wealthy household; and 5, a nonserious illness in a poor household. In addition, all involve a known remedy. All three of these are associated with trying the least expensive alternative to see if it will work (cost-ordered pattern of resorting to treatment). The expectation here is that economic limitations will constrain the treatment choices of the less wealthy who are faced with serious illnesses so that their pattern of choice will be similar to that of the more wealthy who are faced with nonserious illnesses. It would be expected, for example, in cases where physicians (generally the most expensive alternative) are at some point used, that the number of prior treatment actions taken (such as, curer, *practicante*) would be greater among the less wealthy than among the more wealthy.

These two patterns of treatment choices—probability-of-cure ordered, and cost ordered—are in fact evident in the data from the paired comparison interviews, particularly when we examine the variation that occurred between informants of markedly different economic status. One, who is among the poorest in town, repeatedly stressed that alternatives involving substantial expense, particularly those involving physicians, would be used only after all other locally available means had failed. As a general rule he explained that "we always look for where they charge least." In contrast, a second informant, whose household is among the wealthiest in the interview sample, explained that with serious illness "it's necessary to see a *médico*—it doesn't matter what it costs." However, in the majority of households between these wealth extremes either ordering may occur, depending upon the gravity of the illness.

A MODEL OF TREATMENT
DECISION MAKING

The remainder of this chapter is devoted to the presentation and verification of a model of treatment decisions in Pichátaro, constructed on the basis of the interview materials described in the preceding section. It is intended as a formal, concise description of these data. The model specifies the relevant considerations in making treatment choices, as reported by informants, and the ways in which specific combinations of considerations lead to decisions to follow one, rather than several other, courses of action. Table 6.4, which deals with the initial choice of treatment, is the first portion of this model. The reader may find it helpful to refer occasionally to this table during the description that follows. A more detailed discussion of the method of representation, the decision table, may be found in Appendix C.

The model is presented in the form of a decision table. Decision tables (Pollack et al. 1971; see also Miller and Johnson-Laird 1976:281–290) specify: 1. the conditions (considerations) affecting choices;[8] 2. the actions that may be chosen; and 3. the rules of choice, that is, the particular combinations of conditions that lead to each action. The model represented in Table 6.4 includes four conditions and nine rules, or paths, defining the various states of some or all of these conditions. Each path (read vertically) specifies the most probable choice of treatment when a particular combination of conditions exists. Each path may be regarded as a hypothesis concerning the use of a given alternative. If we score actual cases according to each relevant condition in the table, we can test the accuracy of the model in accounting for observed treatment choices. As the initial source of treatment the model defines two paths that lead to the choice of self-treatment, three leading to the choice of a traditional curer, three leading to the choice of a local *practicante,* and one leading to the selection of a physician.

We will begin by considering each condition incorporated into the model and how the decision maker determines its relevant states. These are the four considerations that emerged from the paired comparison interviews.

Gravity

The judged gravity or seriousness of an illness is a primary consideration in treatment decisions. Chapter Three discussed how Pichatareños normally distinguish three main levels of gravity. That is, while the gravity of an illness might ideally be conceived of as a continuous attribute, it appears that the task of dealing with it conceptually is simplified by classification into a small number of classes. People then regard illnesses within the same class as more or less equivalent in gravity. Accordingly, three levels of gravity are specified in the model.

1. Nonserious: The first level corresponds to what is commonly described as "small," "brief," or "simple" illness. These terms are used more or less equivalently to describe nonserious illnesses of short duration. An illness episode that allowed normal activities to continue, or that did not involve an interruption of daily routine for more than a day or two, would probably be judged as of this level of gravity. Not surprisingly, nonserious illnesses are the most frequent type in Pichátaro. The following are examples of symptoms which informants rated as indicative of nonserious illnesses (see Chapter Three): headache, sore throat, toothache, runny nose, aching joints, slightly elevated temperature, stomachache, and dizziness.

2. Moderately serious: Illnesses that more substantially interrupt daily activities by requiring one to remain in bed, that last longer than a few days, and especially those that resist initial treatment attempts, are referred to as "more complicated," "stronger,"

or "regular." These terms describe the second level of gravity. Often, common illnesses such as *gripa* ('cold,' 'flu'), appearing initially with symptoms usually characteristic of later stages of prolonged episodes (such as high temperature or bleeding from the nose), will be described thus. Illnesses at this level of gravity are not regarded as life threatening, although they might become so if not attended to. Informants rated the following symptoms, among others, as indicative of the second level of gravity: backache ("aching lungs"), moderate fever, mild pains in the chest, bloody stool, swelling in the throat, sharp earache, and coughing up phlegm. About one-third of the episodes in the case history materials reached this level of gravity.

3. Grave: The principal distinction between illnesses of the second and third levels of gravity is that the latter constitute potential threats to life. They may involve excessive pain and discomfort, as well as considerable functional impairment. People described such illnesses as "grave," "dangerous," or "heavy." Some symptoms of grave illness include: breathing difficulty, high fever, unconsciousness, heavy bleeding, heart pains, and inability to speak. Overall, illnesses of this seriousness are relatively infrequent.

Pichatareños assessments of gravity take into account the interaction between the severity of the illness and the resistance of the victim. The very old, young children, and especially infants are considered to lack resistance, and their illnesses almost always evoke considerable concern. People believe that certain constitutional factors are related to resistance. For example, some are said to have "damaged blood" (resulting from a poor diet), which lowers their resistance, or to have blood which more easily "carries" illness. Thus, the "same" illness, in terms of its symptoms, could represent different levels of gravity in two different individuals, if for one of the above reasons one of them lacked resistance.

In judgments of the gravity of an illness, certain symptoms are highly salient. Body temperature is directly related to assessments of seriousness; unusually high fever is always regarded as grave. With *gripa,* perhaps the most common illness in Pichátaro, the seriousness attributed to a particular episode varies directly with the level of *calentura* ("temperature") detected. Any illness which restricts or makes more difficult vital body functions, such as breathing and eating, is regarded as serious. Chest pains, particularly "pains in the heart," are always taken to indicate a serious condition. Any illness or injury that involves bleeding is also considered to be moderately serious or grave, depending upon the loss of blood. Some Pichatareños (although there is no consensus on this) consider blood to be irreplaceable and nonregenerating; thus any significant loss means reduced vitality and strength for life. Unconsciousness is, in terms of gravity, believed second only to death itself.

The actual or anticipated duration of the illness is another consideration relevant to how people determine its seriousness. Most illnesses, except those involving fairly extreme symptoms at the onset, are initially regarded as nonserious. However, if a given condition persists, and especially if it resists initial treatment attempts, it is then likely to be regarded as more serious—as having more "strength" than was initially apparent.

Ultimately, the gravity that people attribute to an illness episode depends upon the extent to which they believe life is endangered. For additional discussion of how symptoms are evaluated in judgments of gravity, see Chapter Three.

Knowledge of a Home Remedy

The second consideration that treatment decisions sometimes depend upon is whether or not a home remedy is known for the particular type of illness. This is the only significant constraint on self-treatment. In Table 6.4, a "yes" indicates that a remedy is known within the household and available without resort to a curing specialist. A "no" indicates that no appropriate remedy is known, or that the treatment necessarily involves the skills and knowledge of some specialist, thus ruling out self-treatment.

One reason that people sometimes do not know an appropriate herbal remedy, in particular, is that those most expert in their use—local folk curers—generally keep their ingredients a secret. One informant explained:

> We have a relative, Doña _____ , who is a curer. Some-
> times we don't know the remedy so we go to her. We have to go to her
> because she doesn't tell us what is in the remedy and keeps it hidden
> to one side while making it. I wish I could find out!

In most situations where self-treatment is thought appropriate, a home remedy is known and administered. Occasionally, however, an illness occurs for which neither household members nor neighbors and relatives with whom the problem is discussed know a remedy that can be used with any confidence. In some households a particular type of illness may so often defy home treatment that people feel "we don't know this illness well." In such cases, it becomes necessary to consult a curing specialist; whether this will be a *practicante* or a folk curer depends primarily upon the consideration of faith.

Faith

The third consideration that the model specifies as relevant to choices of treatment is the person's estimate of the potential effectiveness of folk versus medical treatment and remedies in curing the particular illness. This consideration, spoken of as "faith" *(fe),* is illustrated in the following comments:

> . . . You can go to the nurses to see if they can help you. They can
> cure *gripa* faster. But if you have *fe* in the curer and know that she
> can cure the thing, better to go there.

> . . . Now they will go to the *curandera* to see if she can cure it. Often people have more *fe* in the doctor than the curer, but if the doctors can't cure it, they will see if the curer can because she is often able to.

In the first example the informant explains, in effect, that the choice between a *practicante* (the nurse) and a curer will depend upon one's estimate of each alternative's likelihood of providing a cure. The important difference between them is that *practicantes* provide treatment using medical remedies, whereas curers use folk remedies. Which will be favored depends largely on the particular type of illness involved, and one's past experience in treating it.

In the second example, the informant comments that doctors are often thought to offer a high likelihood of cure—people have more faith in them—but that at times, as suggested here, they are unable to help. In such cases one must reevaluate the situation and decide whether a curer's treatment represents, in this specific case, a higher likelihood of success. Here again, faith becomes a matter of choosing between folk and medical treatment.

In this context the meaning of the term "faith" is narrower than might otherwise be construed. It should not be taken here to indicate an enduring commitment to one or the other system of treatment or to a particular practitioner, nor should it be understood to imply any sort of mysticism or religiosity (as in faith healing) or belief with no need of validation. What faith does denote, in relation to illness treatment decisions, is a subjective judgment of the relative probability of cure associated with each of the two forms of treatment. Accordingly, in Table 6.4 for the condition Faith, an F indicates a judgment favoring folk treatment, and an M a judgment favoring medical treatment.

Faith judgments do not depend primarily upon a fixed dichotomy of folk versus medically treatable illnesses, although there are a few illness types which are widely regarded as curable only with folk curing methods. These include *mollera caída* ('fallen fontanel'), *mal de ojo* ('evil eye'), and any illness in which witchcraft is implicated as the cause. In addition, most people agree that medical treatment is not effective for *lastimaduras* ('sprains and bruises'). On the other hand, no illnesses are consistently regarded as curable only with medical treatment (although there is some skepticism about the effectiveness of folk treatment for *fiebre* ['fever'] and a few other grave illnesses). Apart from these special cases, however, people usually agreed that for the majority of illnesses—including all of the most common types—either form of treatment can be effective.

I developed a special interviewing procedure to investigate further the nature of faith judgments. Eleven informants were asked to rank a number of treatment alternatives, including the four principal ones in the model, according to how likely successful treatment would be for each of thirteen different types of illness. People make this type of judgment frequently when talking about illness treatment in less formal contexts: one alternative will be said to be *más cierto* ('more certain,' or 'more sure') than another (see, for example, the response to Situation 1, quoted earlier). The ranking was done separately for each of the following: grippe, fever, swollen glands in the neck, pneumonia, bronchitis, dysentery, vomiting, evil eye, heart illness, bile, fallen fontanel, smallpox, and when the illness type is unknown. Since there were eleven informants and thirteen illness types, a total of 143 separate rankings were created.

Considering all rankings, treatment by a physician received an average rank of 1.5 (highest relative probability of cure); that by a *practicante* averaged 2.6, curer 2.7, and self-treatment 3.2 (lowest relative probability of cure). Physicians consistently ranked quite high. Considering all thirteen illness types, a physician was judged to offer a greater likelihood of cure than a *practicante* in 79% of the rankings, as compared with a curer in 73%. Excluding fallen fontanel and evil eye—both generally considered folk-treatment-only illnesses—a physician was judged as "more certain" than either a curer or a *practicante* in 86% and 94% of the rankings, respectively. Of particular interest are the rankings of curers and *practicantes* relative to each other. Considering all illness types, *practicantes* were rated higher in only 48% of the rankings. Eliminating fallen fontanel and evil eye, they were favored in 57% of the rankings. Both of these are quite close to a 50–50 split between curer and *practicante*. These results show, then, that there is no generally applicable probability-of-cure ordering for these two alternatives, as there are for both the physician and self-treatment alternatives.

These findings are summarized in Figure 6.1. The scale at the top of the figure shows that for most kinds of illness, treatment by a physician is considered to offer the highest likelihood of cure. Self-treatment, on the other hand, is considered to offer the lowest likelihood of producing a cure, relative to the other alternatives. The two remaining alternatives—folk curers and *practicantes*—have no general orderings. The way in which they are depicted in Figure 6.1 is not meant to suggest that they are considered equally likely to

succeed, but rather what is considered the more likely frequently
varies, depending upon the kind of illness and the person's experience with it.

I have said that physicians represented the greatest likelihood of
producing a cure for most illnesses. A few types, mentioned earlier,
are considered curable only with folk remedies. In these exceptional
cases, then, the general faith rank ordering just described doesn't
apply, and a folk curer (or even self-treatment) is judged to offer
better chances of cure. However, since cases of this type are infrequent, the decision maker usually need not actually reason out
whether a physician's treatment offers the best chances of cure, but
rather may just make the routine assumption that it does. On the
other hand, in choosing between the curer and the *practicante* no
such routine assumption can be made. Here, the person must decide, given the particular circumstances and characteristics of the
case at hand, which of the two is more likely to be effective.[9] Since
the most significant difference between these two alternatives is the
type of remedy involved, the faith judgment again becomes a matter of choosing between folk and medical treatment.

What determines faith preferences with respect to curers and
practicantes? In general, estimates of the effectiveness of one or the
other form of treatment are based on people's own experiences, and
those related by friends and kin, with the particular kind of illness
and the perceived successes and failures of each practitioner in
dealing with it. Since different people have access to different information about past successes, there is a good deal of variation in
opinions about which kind of practitioner is best for a given illness.
Nevertheless, there are some general tendencies in faith judgments:
curers are usually favored for children's and emotion-based illnesses (such as bile), whereas *practicantes* are often preferred for
cold-like illnesses, such as grippe.

As I mentioned earlier, such tendencies do not constitute any
sort of general classification of illness into medically-curable and
folk-curable types. Proponents of this "folk dichotomy" theory (see
Chapter One), notably Erasmus (1952, 1961; see also G. Foster
1958), have suggested that such classifications often develop as a
result of people's long-term observations of the successes and fail-

ures of different treatments for specific illness types. However, psychological research on probability judgments under uncertainty provides good reason to believe that such dichotomies are unlikely to develop. Tversky and Kahneman (1974) have found that in estimating the probability of a given event, people use a judgmental heuristic called *availability:* they base their estimates on past occurrences which come most easily to mind. In particular, recent occurrences of an event are more available than earlier ones, and thus influence the probability estimate to a much greater degree. Therefore, it is reasonable to expect that the most important determinant of faith in a given instance will be recollections of what was successful the last time (or at most the last few times) a similar illness occurred, regardless of the frequency of successful cures associated with a given form of treatment over the long run. If this view is correct, one would expect faith judgments to shift frequently from one illness episode to the next. This is indeed the case in Pichátaro, as examples included later in the chapter will illustrate.[10]

Accessibility (Cost and Transportation)

Of the four alternatives included in the model, treatment by a physician is the only one for which cost was consistently cited as a relevant consideration. While all of the alternatives involve some cost, only with the physician is this regularly problematic. Similarly, the availability of transportation is a relevant consideration in the decision to consult a physician, and was cited as such in the interviews, since the nearest are in Pátzcuaro. Since both of these constraints must be met before a physician may be consulted, the physician alternative is not equally accessible at all times or for all people. Therefore, in Table 6.4 for the condition Accessibility, a "yes" indicates that sufficient funds to meet the expected costs of the visit to a doctor, and suitable transportation, are available. A "no" indicates that either or both of these are presently not available, thus ruling out this alternative.

Curers and *practicantes* are for practical purposes equally accessible to almost everyone in Pichátaro. The costs involved are moderate by local standards and usually not problematic; for those unable to pay at the time, most curers and *practicantes* will provide treatment on credit or in exchange for various goods. In contrast, it is well known that physicians (including the Pátzcuaro Health Center) demand payment at the time of treatment. Although their charges are thought roughly proportional to the gravity of the illness, they are viewed as largely unpredictable. There is in fact a high variance in what physicians charge from one visit to the next, and people feel that they must have enough money with them to cover all reasonable contingencies. A visit to a doctor is said to cost "at least" two hundred and fifty pesos—equivalent to earnings from six days' local wage labor—and at times a thousand pesos or more.

There are several ways people can obtain the necessary funds. A few households are sufficiently wealthy to have enough cash on hand to cover the cost immediately. For most, however, an attempt must be made to raise the money. The methods of doing so, in their order of preference, are: obtain an unsecured loan; sell an animal; or pledge a plot of land or one's house. Unsecured loans are most often obtained from kin and *compadres,* and are preferred means of raising money, since no interest is expected upon repayment (which may be considerably delayed). In fact, *compadrazgo* ties are often made with wealthier persons specifically for the purposes of having such support in times of need. Persons with regular incomes, such as school teachers (and, for a time, visiting anthropologists!), are sometimes approached for loans in these situations. If it is not possible to obtain an unsecured loan, an animal may be sold. There is usually a ready market for pigs, sheep, and other livestock in Pichátaro, and a common strategy for obtaining several hundred pesos quickly is to arrange for the sale of an animal. Quick sales may also be made to livestock dealers in Pátzcuaro. The least preferred means of obtaining funds is through loans from a local moneylender. A few such persons in town will make loans secured by agricultural land, one's house, or part of one's house lot. Usually this is an act of desperation in cases involving heavy expenses, as moneylenders charge substantial interest (about 25% per month), and the land or house which is pledged as security is often lost unless the loan can be repaid quickly.

One other strategy exists. A few people explained that they occasionally go to a physician and appeal to his or her compassion, asking that treatment be provided even though they don't have enough money to make full payment. Apparently this can be successful, at least with certain doctors in Pátzcuaro. I was told that this is most effective if one's oldest, most tattered clothing is worn during the visit.

Even in situations where enough money can be raised, treatment by physicians may be delayed, or not occur at all, because transportation from town is not available. The buses do not run with great frequency or at night, and one or both of the town's taxis may be out of order. (The cost of transportation is also a consideration: ill persons rarely, if ever, make a journey alone, and the cost of several round-trip fares may add significantly to the cost of a physician's treatment.) In such cases another local treatment alternative must be used, if for no other purpose than to "calm" the illness. Sometimes very ill persons feel too weak to attempt the trip. Or there may be hesitancy to expose those gravely ill to dangerous "airs" by taking them outdoors. Ironically then, people are sometimes *too* ill to be treated by a physician, and so people resort to another alternative out of necessity.

The General Principles of Treatment Decision Making

Before introducing the specifics of the model of treatment decision making, it may be useful to review briefly the general principles underlying it, and the interrelationships between the four primary considerations I have described. Figure 6.1 depicts the relationship between two of these considerations, faith and cost (the primary component of accessibility). What is apparent here is that the two orderings (both derived from informants' rankings) are parallel: the alternative judged to offer the highest likelihood of cure (a physician) is also the most expensive; that judged least likely to result in a cure (self-treatment) is also the cheapest. The curer and *practicante* alternatives are intermediate and of approximately the same cost. (Again, they are not considered equally likely to result in a cure, but rather, their relative ordering depends upon

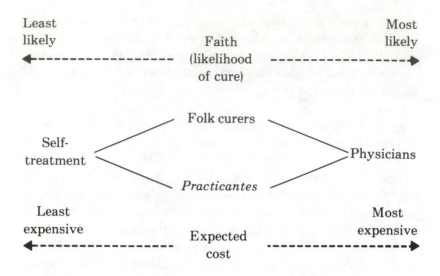

Figure 6.1.   **Faith and Cost Rank Orderings for Most Illness Types**

a faith judgment, and therefore may vary from one situation to the next.)

The judged gravity of the illness is the primary determinant of the order in which the different alternatives will be used. As I described earlier, there are two basic orderings—probability-of-cure ordered, and cost ordered. For nonserious illnesses, the alternatives are ordered on the basis of estimated cost, and the strategy is to avoid as much expense as possible by trying the least costly alternative first—almost always self-treatment. If the illness continues (but is still not considered grave) a *practicante* or folk curer will be consulted. Since these are of approximately equal cost, the one people will choose depends upon a faith judgment: which one is more likely to cure it? A physician, the most expensive alternative, would be used only as a last resort in cases of illness judged not grave. Thus, in Figure 6.1, choices proceed from left to right for nonserious illnesses.

For grave illnesses, on the other hand, the alternatives are ordered on the basis of probability of cure. People ideally first choose the alternative they believe is most likely to cure the illness, regardless of the cost. This, in most cases, is a physician. A generally less certain alternative, such as a curer, would then be tried only after physicians had been unable to achieve a cure.

Moderately serious illnesses, since they are not yet considered life threatening, are generally associated with a cost-ordered sequence of treatment choices. A *practicante,* however, is likely to be chosen initially if people's faith favors medical remedies.

Obviously, there are exceptions to these two ideal patterns, occurring most frequently when the means are not available to realize a particular choice. For example, in situations where a probability-of-cure ordering is in effect, consultation with a physician may not be possible because of cost or transportation constraints. Similarly, in situations of cost ordering, self-treatment may not be possible because an appropriate remedy is unknown or unavailable. In such a case, people would use the next-cheapest alternative, either a curer or a *practicante.* Also, the ordering people follow up to a given point in an illness episode may change if they believe the gravity of the illness is changing.

In essence, then, the model incorporates some basic assumptions concerning what sources of treatment people prefer in different situations and then specifies considerations that may lead to their choosing less preferred alternatives. First I will describe the model and then test it with data from a series of actual illness episodes.

The Initial Choice of Treatment

The nine rules included in Table 6.4 specify when each of the four considerations I described constitutes a relevant consideration, and to what treatment alternative specific configurations of these lead. The rules read vertically, and may be thought of as if-then statements. For example, Rule 1 reads: "*If* an illness is initially judged to be nonserious, *and* an appropriate home remedy is known, *then* self-treatment will be the initial treatment chosen." No value is given for faith or accessibility because, in the situation defined by Rule 1, these are not relevant considerations. That is, since self-treatment may involve use of either folk or medical remedies, no determination of the relative effectiveness of one over the other need precede the choice of this alternative. Since the remedies

Table 6.4. **Decision Table for Initial Choice of Treatment**

Rules:	1	2	3	4	5	6	7	8	9
Conditions									
Gravity[a]	1	1	1	2	2	2	3	3	3
Known home remedy[b]	Y	N	N	Y	N				
Faith[c]		F	M	(F)	F	M	F	M	(M)
Accessibility[d]								N	Y
Choices									
Self-treatment	X			X					
Curer		X			X	X			
Practicante			X			X		X	
Physician									X

[a] 1 = Nonserious; 2 = Moderately serious; 3 = Grave.
[b] Y = Yes; N = No.
[c] F = Favors folk treatment; M = Favors medical treatment.
[d] Y = Money and transportation available; N = Either money or transportation not available.

involved cost little or are simply gathered (in the case of herbal remedies), cost (accessibility) is not an issue.

Rules 2 and 3 specify what choices will be made for nonserious illnesses when no home remedy is known. Here the person must estimate whether folk or medical treatment offers the higher likelihood of cure for the particular illness (a faith judgment): if this judgment favors folk treatment, a curer will be the initial choice (Rule 2); if it favors medical treatment, a *practicante* will be chosen (Rule 3). Again, the accessibility consideration is not a determining factor, since the cost associated with these two alternatives is rarely problematic and is approximately the same for both.

In moderately serious illness, if an appropriate home remedy is known, self-treatment will be chosen unless medical treatment is specifically judged to offer a higher likelihood of cure (Rule 4). The parentheses in Rule 4 are a notational convention designating an implicit judgment. They indicate that a faith evaluation does not routinely occur in this situation, but if it should, its outcome must be in favor of folk treatment; otherwise, by Rule 6, a *practicante* will be chosen.[11] By rule 5, if no home remedy is known, and folk treatment is considered to offer the best chance of cure, a folk curer will be consulted.[12]

The last three rules in Table 6.4 deal with the choice of treatment in the case of illnesses initially judged to be grave. Here, the model assumes a probability-of-cure based preference ordering and accessibility thus becomes a highly relevant consideration. By Rule 9, in grave illnesses, in which sufficient funds are available to meet the expected cost of a visit to a doctor, and suitable transportation can be arranged, the choice will be a physician. Rule 9 also contains an implicit judgment. As I mentioned earlier, a physician's treatment is routinely assumed to offer the highest probability of cure, except in the few special cases of illnesses thought curable only through folk treatment. Thus in these situations a faith evaluation usually would not occur. If it were to occur, however, its outcome would favor medical treatment or else, by Rule 7, a curer would be chosen. Finally, by Rule 8, if access to a physician's treatment is not possible because of cost or transportation constraints, and the faith judgment favors medical treatment, a *practicante* will be chosen as a kind of "poor man's doctor."

Subsequent Choices of Treatment

There are frequently instances in which a given treatment fails to result in a cure, and some other alternative must then be selected. Of all the treatment choices to be accounted for in the case history data (see Table 6.2), about one-third are such subsequent choices. Table 6.5 completes the model of treatment decision making by specifying what considerations people use in making these choices. Since the preceding choice is an important consideration in deciding what alternative to use next, this is incorporated into the table along with three of the same considerations found in Table 6.4.

The length of time people try a given treatment before it is considered a failure varies a good deal, but in general the less serious an illness, the longer the period before they choose a new alternative. Folk remedies are usually expected to cure more slowly than medical remedies: at times one hears of "successful" cures using folk remedies that took a month to achieve. In contrast, people expect treatments using medical remedies, and especially physicians' treatments, to result in a reduction in symptoms almost at once,

Table 6.5.   **Decision Table for Subsequent Choices of Treatment**

Rules:	1	2	3	4	5	6	7	8	9	10	11
Conditions											
Preceding Choice[a]	ST	ST	ST	ST	C-P	C-P	C	P	Dr	Dr	Dr
Current Gravity[b]		1-2	3	3	1	2-3	2-3	2-3			
Faith[c]	F	M	M	(M)					F		M
Accessibility[d]			N	Y		Y	N	N		N	Y
Choices											
Self-treatment					X						
Curer	X							X	X	X	
Practicante		X	X				X				
Physician				X		X					X

[a] ST = Self-treatment; C = Curer; P = *Practicante;* Dr = Physician.

[b] 1 = Nonserious; 2 = Moderately serious; 3 = Grave.

[c] F = Favors folk treatment; M = Favors medical treatment.

[d] Y = Money and transportation available; N = Either money or transportation not currently available.

and certainly within a few days. Many times recommended return visits are not made, or medications not continued, because the initial medication did not produce a marked improvement in the patient, who considers the treatment to have failed. In almost all cases, people use alternatives sequentially rather than concurrently. The only significant exception is that self-treatment is sometimes continued even after resort to another alternative.

Subsequent choices often involve a reevaluation of relevant conditions. In particular, faith judgments may change in the light of the current lack of success of a given type of treatment, and changes in the judged gravity of the illness may result in a shift from one ordering of alternatives to the other.

Rules 1 through 4 of Table 6.5 depict the basis upon which people make subsequent choices following unsuccessful home treatment. If they now consider the illness grave, and sufficient money and transportation are available, they will consult a physician (Rule 4), provided there is no reason to believe that folk treatment offers a better chance of cure. If the accessibility constraint cannot be met, and the faith judgment favors medical treatment, people will resort to a *practicante* (Rule 3). If, following self-treatment, they think that folk treatment offers the highest likelihood of success, they will consult a curer regardless of the apparent gravity of the illness (Rule 1). By Rule 2, if the illness is judged not grave and faith favors medical treatment, people will again choose a *practicante*.

In those cases in which people consulted a curer unable to achieve a cure, their subsequent choice of treatment will be governed by the considerations shown in Rules 5 through 7. If they now consider the illness nonserious, home treatment will be given (Rule 5). Otherwise, the model assumes that because of the ineffectiveness of the curer's treatment, medical remedies will now be favored as offering the best prospects for cure. Accordingly, if the illness is moderately serious or grave, and the means are available, a physician will be consulted (Rule 6); if the means are lacking, a *practicante* will be chosen (Rule 7).

In those cases in which a *practicante* was the initial or preceding choice and was unsuccessful, people do not necessarily rule out medical treatment. It is said that physicians have better and "stronger" medicines than *practicantes,* and are often able to cure an illness that has resisted the latter's remedies. As shown, again in Rule 6, if the illness is now considered moderately serious or grave, and money and transportation are available, a physician will be used. If the means are not available a curer will be consulted (Rule 8), since this is the only other option. If the illness is thought non-serious (Rule 5), a person would administer self-treatment.

The last possibility is that the person's preceding action involved resort to a physician, in which case he will choose any subsequent treatment according to Rules 9 through 11. Basically the decision that must be made is whether to continue medical treatment with another doctor, or turn to a folk-curing specialist. This will be governed by the person's reassessment of his faith in medical treatment, and the continued availability of the money to pay for the physician's treatment. If his faith in medical treatment remains greater, and the means are still available, another physician— perhaps a specialist (see Chapter Five)—will be consulted (Rule 11). If a person's faith continues to favor medical treatment but the money has run out (Rule 10), or if he feels that folk treatment offers a higher probability of cure, the doctor(s)' having failed (Rule 9), he will consult a curer. A *practicante* is not considered in this case since, it is reasoned, if a doctor has been unable to cure the illness, the *practicante,* with less potent remedies, would not be able to either.

Some Examples of Treatment Choice

To make more concrete how people choose treatment, as represented in the model, I will describe a series of illness case histories. They are from two households that vary substantially in terms of composition and economic resources; to provide some control for the comparison, both sets of illnesses involve young children.

The first three cases involve the same male infant (Enrique), who at the time case collection began was five months old. He and his parents reside with his father's maternal grandparents, who are in their seventies. Enrique's father, who was eighteen years old at the time, is an artisan who carves wooden figures and frames for sale to dealers in Pátzcuaro and Quiroga. He and his wife each completed a little over three years of schooling. Enrique is their first child. On a wealth ranking of households in the case collection sample (see Appendix A) this household rated in the upper one-third in terms of overall economic resources. The grandfather is a farmer with above-average land holdings. The infant had been ill only once prior to the case collection period, a short-lived case of *mollera caída* that was treated at home by the grandmother.

In February, 1976, Enrique developed a case of *la gripa* ('cold,' 'flu'), which lasted for about seven days. He had an above normal temperature, was coughing, and had a runny nose. His parents attributed his illness to a "change of weather." The first day he showed these symptoms they applied a home remedy—a locally bought cream that the family often uses for this type of illness. On the second day his illness continued, the home treatment having had no effect thus far. His mother explained that they were uncertain what was wrong with their child, and that they had become considerably worried over it, especially considering Enrique's age. As she put it, *"niños son delicados"* ('children are frail'). Although she did not express it, it is probable that they feared the illness would become even more serious. Since Enrique is their first and only child this no doubt added to their judgment of the illness's gravity. Thus on the second day the decision was made to take him to a private-practice physician in Pátzcuaro. There he received an injection and a liquid medication, at a total cost (exclusive of transportation) of 111 pesos. The medication was continued on the third and fourth days, but the symptoms persisted. On the fifth and sixth days of the illness Enrique was taken to a local curer who applied herbal remedies to the child's body. By the seventh day the symptoms were diminishing, and soon after he was considered well. His mother, interviewed the following day, attributed his recovery to the curer's treatment. The curer, her grandmother, collected ten pesos for the treatment.

Approximately five weeks later Enrique again became ill, this time with a mild case of *calentura* ('temperature'). This was essentially the same type of illness as on the previous occasion, although this time it was less serious and involved only a mild fever, and none of the other symptoms. On the first day he was sick his mother treated him with another store-bought remedy. He showed no improvement on the second day, and so was taken to the same curer as in the previous case. His mother stated that injections and other *remedios médicos* "can't cure this illness," and that they now had more "faith" in the curer and her remedies. The infant was well the next day.

One month after the second episode, Enrique experienced a third illness which persisted for over ten days. His parents believed that it came about from a fright or scare that the child had suffered, resulting in *la bilis* ('bile'). The symptoms of this were diarrhea and later, occasional vomiting. On the first day the symptoms were present his mother gave him some pills and herbal remedies. By the third day it became apparent that the home treatment was ineffective, and Enrique was taken again to the same curer, where he was given more herbal remedies. On the fourth through sixth days there was no substantial change in what were now considered rather severe symptoms. On the seventh day of the illness he was taken to Pátzcuaro for treatment by a private physician. The symptoms began to diminish the following day, and after three more days the child was considered well.

In the first episode, the initial action taken was home treatment.

The illness was at this point not considered grave, and a home remedy was known, therefore Rule 6.4–4 (Table 6.4, Rule 4) correctly indicates that home treatment would be chosen. By the second day, there is evidence that Enrique's parents were beginning to doubt their ability to handle the illness themselves, and his extremely young age contributed to the assessment of seriousness. From records of earlier cases of *gripa* in this household we knew that medical treatment had been used successfully a number of times, so in this instance we are justified in assuming that folk treatment was not regarded as offering a better chance of cure. Therefore Rule 6.5–4 correctly accounts for the choice of a physician's treatment. There is no direct a priori evidence that the money to do so was in fact available (as specified by the model); in this case we must assume that it was since the household is above the median wealth rank. On the third and fourth days the persistence of the illness in spite of the physician's treatment led Enrique's parents to reassess their faith in the effectiveness of medical treatment in curing *gripa*. Then, as Rule 6.5–9 suggests would occur, the infant was taken to a curer.

The second illness is a good illustration of how substantial the effect of recent outcomes can be for faith judgments. Initially, as in most cases, home treatment was administered (Rule 6.4–1). When Enrique's mother determined on the second day that other treatment should be sought, her faith judgment now clearly favored herbal remedies (on the basis of what succeeded the last time a similar illness occurred), and (by Rule 6.5–1) the illness was referred to the curer.

The last episode also began, as usual, with home treatment (Rule 6.4–4). Since the illness continued, other treatment was considered. Recalling that a curer had been successful in treating Enrique on two previous occasions, and medical remedies had never, in his parents' view, been of help to him, they now regarded folk treatment as offering the highest probability of cure in this instance as well. Apart from this, curers are generally considered to be "good" with this type of illness. Therefore, again by Rule 6.5–1, a curer was consulted. Now, however, her treatment seemed to have no effect, and the illness appeared to be continuing on a dangerous course. A physician was at this point consulted (Rule 6.5–6), reflecting yet another change in their estimate of the efficacy of medical versus folk treatment. Again we may consider the household's relatively high economic standing as indirect evidence that they had the means available to consult a physician.

The pattern that emerges from these three illness episodes is that once the illness comes to be viewed as serious, it is referred to whatever alternative is thought to offer the highest relative probability of successful treatment. Cost is a much less important consideration. It is informative now to compare the above cases with the following two episodes from a much poorer household. Both of the cases involve a one-year-old girl, who we will call Josefina. Her father is a landless laborer who has few possessions other than his house. He and his wife have a son and two other daughters. This household was rated among the poorest one-fifth in the sample.

Josefina's first illness, simply termed *vómito* ('vomiting') by her mother, persisted for almost three weeks. During this time the child ate little, had a high temperature, and vomited intermittently. At the onset her mother described the illness as moderately serious, but as it prolonged and the child continued to eat very little, she came to describe it as very grave. On the first day of the illness Josefina's mother prepared a standard herbal remedy for her, and repeated this treatment for a few days. Despite this the illness continued, and the child was taken to a curer. The curer administered another herbal remedy but was also unable to achieve a cure. Next, the medical post nurse (a *practicante*) was consulted, and medication given. After this treatment the illness persisted for several days, but during this time the symptoms were diminishing and eventually were alleviated. Her mother explained that the girl had not been taken to a physician in Pátzcuaro because there was simply not enough money to do so. The total expenditure on the treatment was twenty-five pesos.

About two months later Josefina came down with a case of *la gripa* that lasted for over two weeks. For approximately the first week the symptoms were mild and intermittent. Her mother described it as "not very big" and gave the child aspirin tablets purchased at a local store. During the second week, however, the fever became "much stronger," and the parents related that they became very worried, and took Josefina to a *practicante* for an injection. This did not cut the fever, and so at the beginning of the third week she was taken to a physician in Pátzcuaro—after her father was successful in borrowing the money. This treatment finally resulted in a cure, at the cost of around one hundred pesos. Josefina's parents refused to pay the *practicante* anything because she had been unable to effect a cure.

In contrast with the pattern of treatment choices made during Enrique's illness, Josefina's parents always resorted to the least costly alternatives. In her first illness they began treatment with household remedies, since the illness was initially not grave and a remedy was known (Rule 6.4–4). The next choice, when the illness failed to respond to home treatment, was a curer. This is as Rule 6.5–1 indicates, since folk treatment is generally thought, by Josefina's parents and by most Pichatareños, to be more effective for this type of illness. Following the curer's lack of success the parents chose a *practicante* (Rule 6.5–7) because the means were not available to take the child to a physician.

The second illness began as nonserious and received home treatment (Rule 6.4–1). When it came to be considered grave in the second week, a *practicante,* rather than a physician, was consulted because of the cost constraint (Rule 6.5–3). Medical treatment is usually favored for *la gripa,* and had been used in this household in the past, thus the choice of a *practicante* rather than a curer. Only when no other alternative was left did they turn to a doctor (Rule 6.5–6). This accords with our finding that in poorer households people will not consult physicians until either a *practicante* or a curer, or in some cases both, have been shown to offer no possibility of a lower-cost cure. Josefina's illnesses illustrate how economic limitations in poorer households constrain choices. In this case, the pattern is basically cost-ordered, even in serious illness.

TESTING THE MODEL

The model of treatment decision making that I have presented may be considered as a series of hypotheses, derived from informants' statements on the conditions under which they choose different treatment alternatives. We will test these utilization rules against a body of illness case history data to determine the extent to which the model is capable of accounting for actual treatment choices.

Although I briefly summarized the case history materials at the beginning of this chapter (and in Chapter Three), and illustrative cases have occasionally been taken from them, I must emphasize that methodologically they constitute data completely independent from that used to generate the model, and may therefore serve as a valid test of it. As shown in Table 6.2, a total of 489 treatment choices were made. The number of choices is greater than the number of cases (323) because over a third of the illnesses involved two or more treatment alternatives, and accordingly present more than a single choice.

The major obstacle to be overcome in making this test was the specification of the conditions that existed leading up to a given treatment choice, independent of the a posteriori evidence provided by the knowledge of the eventual choice. For example, in a case in which a physician was used, we cannot specify with certainty that enough money was available immediately prior to that action, short of the circular evidence that there must have been, since people did in fact make that choice. A subjective element was thus inevitable in the scoring of some cases on the conditions in the model, although I made considerable attempts to minimize it as much as possible. Where this was potentially a problem, specific criteria were set to guide the testing. In cases occurring in households below the median wealth rank, a choice of physician's treatment would be scored as accounted for incorrectly unless a curer or *practicante* were consulted first. This is in accord with the cost-ordered pattern assumed to be in effect in these cases. Similarly, for households above the median wealth rank, I assumed the economic means were available in those situations in which the conditions otherwise indicated the choice of a physician (as in Enrique's illness described earlier).

Other data also helped to minimize subjectivity in the scoring of the conditions "faith" and "known home remedy." From each household in the sample we obtained brief descriptions of past illnesses that had occurred before the case collection period. These data are not necessarily complete, but they do provide information on what illnesses are well known in a given household, and to what extent they have been cured with the different types of treatment in the past. This record is most complete for recent illnesses, which is fortunate since the outcomes of these episodes are likely to be most important in making the faith judgments in the test cases. For example, in a case where a curer was consulted for an illness that might plausibly have been taken to a *practicante,* and there was no explicit statement of greater faith in folk treatment, I could check the record for the most recent past case of the same kind of illness in that household. If it had been successfully treated by a curer on that occasion, I could reasonably assume that the faith judgment favored this type of treatment in the present case. On the other hand, if the previous cure had involved a *practicante,* there would be no a priori basis in the test case to assume greater faith in herbal remedies, and the model would be scored as failing to account for the observed choice. By and large, any errors that these procedures introduced into the testing would tend to be conservative errors. That is, if they do bias the results, it is in the direction of unnecessarily scoring the model as failing to account for a given choice, rather than in the direction of exaggerating its success rate.

Most often, of course, test episodes were scored on the basis of data in the case history. When each case was collected, informants were asked about the situation which led up to their choice of treatment, why they had not chosen other alternatives, and what further actions they were considering if the illness continued. The considerations that people most often cited in explaining and justifying their choices were, as expected, those that are incorporated in the model.

Table 6.6 presents the results of the test. The figures in the totals column represent the number of treatment choice situations that were characterized by the conditions defined by the given rule. For example, there were 157 situations that were as defined by Rule 6.4–1, and all of these led to self-treatment, as the rule would indicate. If we examine the results for Rule 6.4–6, however, while the conditions of twenty-nine treatment choices were as this rule

Table 6.6. **Test Results**

		Alternative chosen					
Table	Rule	Self-treatment	Curer	Practicante	Physician	Totals	Percentage correct
6.4	1	157				157	
	2		4			4	
	3			5		5	
	4	67			(1)	68	
	5		8			8	
	6	(2)		20	(7)	29	
	7		8			8	
	8		(2)	4	(2)	8	
	9			(2)	11	13	
						300	94.7
6.5	1	19				19	
	2		(1)	28	(6)	35	
	3		(3)	6		9	
	4			(2)	22	24	
	5	3	(1)			4	
	6	(2)	(2)	(1)	24	29	
	7	(1)		3	(2)	6	
	8		2	(1)		3	
	9	(1)	7			8	
	10					0	
	11				7	7	
						144	84.0
Subtotal						444	91.2
Not covered						18	
Insufficient data						27	
Total						489	

specifies, in only twenty was the predicted alternative, a *practicante,* actually chosen. In two cases, self-treatment was selected, and in seven instances a physician was consulted. Those choices that the model fails to account for are included in parentheses.

Overall, the model correctly accounts for 91% of the choices included in the test.[13] Its accuracy is highest for initial choices (94.7%), and somewhat lower (84%) with subsequent choices. In particular, it is less accurate in dealing with some choices following treatment by curers and *practicantes* (Rules 6.5–7 and 6.5–8), although these represent relatively few cases and do not seem to indicate any systematic defect in the model. Rules 6.4–1 and 6.4–4, both leading to self-treatment, together constitute half of all choices included in the test, and since they represent a largely routine initial response to illness, we can more easily account for these choices. If they are removed from consideration, the model still correctly accounts for 82.6% of the remaining choices, in which we may assume more active decision making.

These results provide strong evidence for the basic validity of the model, and for the contention that the considerations and assumptions embodied in it represent important aspects of how people actually make these choices. It appears, then, that there are significant regularities in the ways Pichatareños use different treatment alternatives, and to a considerable degree we may anticipate their choices.

In the final chapter we shall review these findings and consider their implications for an overall understanding of medical choice in Pichátaro.

7

Medical Choice in Pichátaro

The central aim of this study has been to describe in a systematic way the rationale underlying how Pichatareños make illness treatment decisions. On the basis of the test results, it seems fair to conclude that this attempt has generally succeeded. Not only have we accounted for a high proportion of the data but we have also obtained specific knowledge of the reasoning behind these choices. This last chapter is concerned with the implications of the study for health-care policy in pluralistic settings like that of Pichátaro. We will also evaluate what the decision-making approach has accomplished and in what directions research might further be pursued. First, however, let us briefly review the findings.

THE CHOICE OF TREATMENT:
A SUMMARY

Four primary criteria are involved in illness treatment decisions in Pichátaro: the gravity or seriousness of the particular illness; whether or not an appropriate home remedy is known for the illness; the faith one has in the effectiveness of folk treatment, as opposed to medical treatment, in alleviating the illness; and the expenses associated with some alternatives and the availability of the resources to meet them.

People tend to select treatment alternatives in accordance with one of two orderings. These orderings are based on two key aspects of the available alternatives: the likelihood that the use of the particular source of treatment would actually result in a cure; and the estimated cost associated with each alternative. In serious illness, when adequate resources are available within the household, alternatives are ordered on the basis of likelihood of cure, and people choose the alternative judged most likely to help. In contrast, in nonserious illness the alternatives are ordered on the basis of expected cost, and people choose the one involving the lowest cost (or the lowest cost of those they have not yet tried). The cost-ordered sequence occurs in this case whether or not people have sufficient funds to cover the cost of a more expensive alternative. In the situation of serious illness in households where resources are scarce (as is quite often the case in Pichátaro), even though people would prefer first to choose highest likelihood of cure, economic limitations constrain their choices in favor of lowest estimated cost, approximating a cost-ordered sequence.

The findings concerning the use of each of the four major treatment alternatives, and the ways in which they fit into the above orderings, may be summarized as follows:

Self-treatment

Self-treatment generally offers the lowest likelihood of cure, relative to the other alternatives, but it is also the least expensive. Since most illnesses in their initial stages are judged to be nonserious, and since this leads to a cost-based preference ordering, self-treatment is by far the most frequent initial response to illness in Pichátaro. In fact, the incidence of illness in most households, particularly those with a number of children, is such that treatment is a generally routine domestic activity. Exceptions to the initial choice of self-treatment occur in two principal ways. When an illness is initially judged as grave, a probability-of-cure preference ordering comes into effect, and people select a treatment alternative offering a higher likelihood of success than self-treatment. Household members will also avoid self-treatment if they have inadequate knowledge of an appropriate remedy.

Folk Curers

Folk curers and *practicantes* fall between self-treatment and physicians in both estimated likelihood of cure and expected cost (on cost they are approximately equal). We found no generally applicable ordering concerning which—folk curer or *practicante*—is more likely to achieve a cure; this varied with the particular case. Since the salient contrast between these two alternatives is the form of treatment, this choice depends upon the person's estimate of the relative likelihood of success using folk versus modern medical treatment. This estimate (one's faith) is based primarily upon one's past experience with the particular type of illness at hand, and often varies between households and from one illness episode to the next.

A prerequisite to all choices of a curer's treatment, then, is that the person must have decided that folk treatment offers a higher likelihood of cure, in terms of his own native standards, than modern medical treatment. People initially choose a curer over self-treatment when they lack knowledge of an appropriate remedy; and over a *practicante* or physician when they judge the illness to be grave, and they think it is more likely to be curable with folk than with medical remedies. In subsequent choices, resort to folk curers occurs most often following unsuccessful self-treatment.

Practicantes

Since *practicantes* and folk curers share two important attributes—both are of modest cost, and both are available locally—the situations in which they are chosen are in many ways similar. Like curers, *practicantes* are most frequently consulted in nonserious illnesses when self-treatment has not been attempted, or else has been tried but found ineffective. When people choose a *practicante,* they assume that medical treatment, in this particular case, affords a higher probability of cure than folk treatment. The situations in which *practicantes* are used for serious illnesses, however, differ from what was found for the curers. While curers represent the culmination of traditional medical practice, *practicantes,* although employing modern medical remedies, are generally considered less skilled and less likely to achieve a cure than a physician. Thus *practicantes* are chosen in grave illnesses when the means are not available to consult a physician, and then only when their remedies are still thought to offer the best chances of success.

Physicians

For most kinds of illness, Pichatareños consider a physician's treatment to offer the highest likelihood of a cure. The expense (this is also the most costly option) and inconvenience of going to a physician for treatment, however, are important constraints. Because the local economy is such that resources in most households are scarce, and often not easily converted to cash, expenditures for a physician's services necessarily must compete with other, often essential, household needs. Accordingly, physicians tend to be used only in certain fairly extreme situations. Initially, if an illness is judged grave—that is, life threatening—a physician will be consulted in most cases, if at all possible. This is in accord with the probability-of-cure preference ordering in such situations. Otherwise, a physician becomes a plausible choice when all other less costly alternatives have proven unsuccessful, or if the illness becomes grave.

The general case may be summarized as follows: of the four decision criteria incorporated in the model, the gravity of the illness is the consideration that determines the overall preference ordering for the treatment alternatives; one's faith serves primarily to establish the relative orderings of the curer and *practicante* alternatives in particular cases; lack of knowledge of a home remedy is a constraint on self-treatment; and accessibility determines whether one will choose treatment by a physician. The formal model—which includes these four criteria and is constructed on the basis of the above assumptions concerning preferred sources of treatment in different situations—was tested with a series of actual illness case histories and found to correctly account for 91% of all treatment choices.

IMPLICATIONS OF THE MODEL

In an earlier discussion (see Chapter Two), I mentioned a current debate concerning the reaction of rural Third World peoples to Western medicine. It has often been observed (see Foster and Anderson 1978:223–262) that such peoples frequently underutilize modern medical services, or at least use them at rates below what health planners might anticipate, as they continue to resort to traditional curing personnel. Two general sorts of explanations for this phenomenon are evident in the literature. One points to the influence of "cultural" factors, such as traditional beliefs about illness and the influence of traditional practitioners, the other to factors of restricted access and exclusion. One of the important advantages of the decision-making approach is that it not only describes the considerations that lead to the use of particular alternatives, but it also describes in equally specific terms why particular alternatives are in given instances *not* chosen (see C. Gladwin 1977:277–286). Let us put this feature of the model to use in evaluating how accurately each of these views portrays treatment decision making in Pichátaro.

The Influence of Traditional Beliefs

A frequent explanation for lower rates of utilization of modern medical resources by rural peoples who also have available traditional (non-Western) treatment alternatives, is that such people's traditional beliefs and cultural inhibitions are inconsistent with, or keep them from realizing the benefits of, Western medical therapy.[1] It is sometimes found, for instance, that people who use Western medical services tend to have characteristics defined as modern (relating to education, literacy, language use and so on). The solution to the problem of increasing the use of such services is then said to lie in the modernization of the population as a whole. Thus, a World Health Organization sponsored study of rural-urban differences in the utilization of health services in Tunisia concluded:

> What seems to have been true for the United States is likely to be even more true in developing countries where education, even of a primary level, is a major force in breaking down reliance upon traditionalistic world views and folk practices. An important function of education is to help individuals cope with their needs by making intelligent use of available social and health services. In countries where traditional health attitudes have been strong and have been

thought by the government to hinder development, educational systems have made special efforts to overcome such attitudes as fatalism or reliance upon folk methods of treatment. Here the aim has been not only to improve the health of the public, but also to motivate a population for participation in a developing economy (Benyoussef and Wessen 1974:302).[2]

Explanations such as these place responsibility for underuse of modern health care services, and accompanying poorer health levels, directly with the people themselves (analogous to some of the implications of the much critiqued "culture of poverty" concept [Valentine 1968]). Such studies advocate modifying the traditional culture and eventually incorporating such peoples into the national economy as the ultimate solution to the problem of providing improved health care.

The findings of the Pichátaro study, on the other hand, present quite a different view in terms of their implications for policy aimed at increasing utilization of modern health care services. It is clear that Pichatareños need little convincing of the effectiveness of modern medical treatment provided by a physician. As we saw in Chapter Six, treatment by a physician is considered, by most people and for most kinds of illnesses, to offer the highest likelihood of cure of the available alternatives. The situations in which traditional curers are considered to offer a higher likelihood of success than a physician (that is, the incidence of Benyoussef and Wessen's "traditional health attitudes") are relatively few and, when one considers the informational bases of these beliefs, not necessarily unreasonable. That is, those illnesses that Pichatareños generally classify as incurable through modern medical treatment are, not by coincidence, also those for which modern medicine in fact has no specific therapy (such as whooping cough and measles); illnesses in which the high likelihood of subsequent reinfection because of often unsanitary living conditions masks the effects of treatment (such as infant diarrhea—a prominent symptom of *mollera caída* and 'evil eye'); or those in which the diagnosis usually implies an earlier failure of medical treatment (such as "witchcraft-caused" illnesses—see Chapter Six).

Most often, Pichatareños do not utilize modern medical treatment more frequently because such services are inaccessible. When a trip to a doctor might cost at least a week's income, and the ill person must be transported on a slow, uncomfortable, and often overcrowded bus for an hour or more, it is not surprising that less expensive and more convenient alternatives are often chosen. Since many households have quite limited resources that must be allocated among a number of essential needs, it seems justifiable, though perhaps regrettable, that illnesses not considered life threatening are found to not warrant the sacrifice of household resources that a physician's treatment would entail.

It is possible, as I mentioned earlier, to trace individual cases through the model and isolate points in the illness episode where a physician's treatment offered a plausible choice—given our understanding of Pichatareños' standards for making such choices—but was in fact not chosen because of one critical consideration. In the case history data there are thirty-eight such instances. Table 7.1 illustrates the frequency with which each of three critical considerations was responsible for the decision not to seek a physician's treatment, when the remaining considerations otherwise rendered this a culturally appropriate choice. These data show that "traditional health attitudes" are a primary factor in no more than one out of five such decisions. Much more frequently the inaccessibility

Table 7.1. **Critical Considerations in Decisions Not to Use a Physician's Treatment**

Reason	*Number*	*Percentage*
Preexisting preference for folk treatment (considered to offer a higher likelihood of cure)	8	21
Accessibility (not enough money available, or no transportation to Pátzcuaro)	22	58
A physician's treatment had just been given but had not achieved a cure	8	21
Total	38	100

of a doctor is responsible for the use of some other alternative. The data also show that the demonstrated inability (in the Pichatareño's view) of a physician's treatment to cure the illness at hand is as often a factor leading to the choice of an alternative treatment as is a preexisting preference for folk treatment methods.

The high price, by local standards, and intermittent availability of a physician's treatment are major determinants of the overall form of the treatment decision-making process in Pichátaro. Not only do these factors sometimes act as constraints in situations where conditions would otherwise indicate the selection of a physician's treatment (see Rules 6.4–8, 6.5–3, 6.5–7, 6.5–8, and 6.5–10 in Tables 6.4 and 6.5, Chapter Six), they are also the principal reasons why only under certain fairly extreme conditions a physician's treatment is considered at all. That is, the frequent implementation of a cost-ordered treatment plan is not a *cause* of lower rates of physician utilization but rather a *consequence* of the relative inaccessibility of such services.

The Role of Traditional Curers

Another frequent explanation for infrequent or delayed use of modern medical services in communities like Pichátaro, is that people's strong allegiance to traditional curing specialists inhibits their use of physicians. This view also contains some significant inaccuracies, applied to the specific case of Pichátaro. The following comments summarize the general understanding of the folk curer's role held by those involved in rural health planning and policy in Mexico:

> The different types of *curanderos* are consulted more frequently in rural areas than are doctors. . . . In practicing their science they make use of their knowledge of ethnomedicine, magic, and, occasionally, modern medicine. . . . They play a very important role in the health of people living in these areas, because the majority of patients consider magic and religion as part of the reason for their being ill, and because rural self-medication is symbolic of prehispanic tradition. . . . Nevertheless, we know too little about these *curanderos* to be able to evaluate their role in health improvement in these areas. . . . (Cañedo 1974:1133).

There is a failure here to distinguish between different treatment options that may, from an informant's point of view, be sharply distinguished (such as *curanderos, practicantes,* and self-treatment). It is also misleading to assert that traditional practices continue because they are "symbolic of prehispanic tradition." Further, the above view considerably exaggerates the significance of magical and supernatural beliefs, both as factors in treatment decisions and as important features of the curer's practice. Presumably these comments refer to such folk illness concepts as evil eye and witchcraft-caused illnesses, which, in Pichátaro at least, represent only a small fraction of all illness episodes, the majority being explained and treated in accordance with more naturalistic principles, as described in Chapter Three.

A much more important point regarding these comments, however, is the a priori assumption that every decision to consult a curer necessarily implies a decision not to consult a physician. To what extent is this true in Pichátaro? Just as it was possible earlier to look at the critical considerations involved in decisions not to use a physician's treatment, here the model allows us to determine which specific alternative was not chosen in each situation when a traditional curer was. That is, it is possible, by tracing individual cases through the model, to specify in each instance a curer was chosen, which remaining alternative represented the next most likely choice had the curer alternative been unavailable.[3] The distribution of these "rejected" alternatives appears in Table 7.2. Here the data show that in less than one-third of all instances in which a curer was chosen was her treatment preferred to a physician's treatment. Further, seven of these cases involved the choice of a

Table 7.2. **Rejected Alternatives to Consulting a Curer**

Instances in which folk curer was selected in preference to:	*Number*	*Percentage*
Self-treatment	1	2
Practicante	39	68
Physician	17	30
Total	57	100

curer following unsuccessful treatment by a physician (Rule 6.5–9); therefore, only 18% of the instances in which a curer was chosen entailed the rejection of a physician's treatment on the basis of a preexisting preference for traditional curers. Thus, in only a relatively few cases can nonuse of physicians by Pichatareños be explained as due to competition from traditional curers.

Conclusions: Access and Marginality

The study findings provide little support for the point of view that it is primarily "cultural" factors, such as traditional beliefs about illness and the presence of folk curing specialists, which account for the less-than-spectacular inroads that Western medicine has made into Pichátaro's health care system. Rather, we see a people with an awareness of, and often as not a genuine enthusiasm for, modern medical treatment, but who are at the same time frequently denied full access to such services. To a considerable degree, in fact, the traditional system of medical beliefs and practices, which remains full and vigorous, and the continuing use of and role for native curers (as well as marginal medical personnel such as the *practicante* Rafael), may be seen as aspects of the community's on-going adaptation to its position of economic and social marginality in relation to the larger Mexican society.

Modern health care services in Mexico are unequally distributed, favoring the urbanite and the regularly employed (see Cañedo 1974), putting rural subsistence farming communities like Pichátaro at a double disadvantage.[4] Most government supported health-care facilities systematically exclude the non-wage earner, and those that do not (such as S.S.A. facilities like the Pátzcuaro Health Center—see Chapter Five) are chronically understaffed and underbudgeted. Despite apparently genuine efforts on the part of the government to provide improved facilities (such as the Ario de Rosales Clinic), it remains true that in seeking modern medical treatment most Pichatareños, most of the time, depend upon the system of health care delivery with which they are least well equipped to cope—the private, fee-for-service physician.

Obviously Pichátaro cannot be claimed to represent all rural Mesoamerica, and even less so marginal rural peoples in general.

Nevertheless, there is some evidence that its orientation to modern medicine is not unique. For example, Beals, in his study of curing choices in two South Indian villages, concluded:

> There is more than a suggestion that in this very conservative village, Western medicine is actually the most expensive and the most prestigious form of medicine. In Namhalli, with its long history of exposure to Western medicine, this is even more true. This casts doubt upon the assumption that rural people maintain a conservative attitude toward Western medicine or a preference for traditional medicine. Rather, it would appear that the preference lies with the most modern and most expensive forms of medicine, but that economic necessity, procrastination, or faulty diagnosis lead to a continuing patronage of alternative systems of medicine (A. Beals 1976:192–194).

These findings are particularly significant since his study is one of the few that have attempted, like the present study, systematically to identify the actual considerations involved in people's decisions about health care.

A study of a rural black community on one of the South Carolina Sea Islands concluded that the local system of "popular" medicine has persisted due to conditions generally analogous to Pichátaro's. The study finds that the system continues in this marginal community because it fills "a serious need caused by the absence or inadequacy of professional medicine largely due to the nature of its 'fee-for-services' system" (Moerman 1974:3). Once again, "popular" or traditional medicine represents one aspect of the community's adaptive response to its position of inequality in relation to the larger society.

When underutilization of modern medical services results less from people's reluctance to use them than from their frequent inaccessibility, it becomes obvious that the solution to health care problems in settings like Pichátaro is not to be found entirely, nor even primarily, within the community itself. Solutions that attempt to deal only with factors internal to the community, such as people's beliefs and attitudes toward modern medicine, cannot lead to significant increases in the use of modern medical services because they do not deal with the most important real world factors constraining such use. In Pichátaro's case, for example, it seems clear that past government policies and national politicoeconomic conditions that have resulted in the overwhelmingly urban concentration of medical resources in Mexico, and regulations that often systematically exclude rural subsistence farmers from using them, have had as much to do with determining the ways in which people in Pichátaro make illness treatment decisions as anything intrinsic to life in Pichátaro itself.

Applied to Pichátaro's case, then, the more traditional views of the factors limiting the utilization of modern medical services by rural Third World peoples do not go very far toward accounting for the actual data. Moreover, the solutions that follow from such explanations seem largely to ignore the most important factors that shape the choices they aim to influence. The primary role of the applied anthropologist, in settings similar to that of Pichátaro, should no longer be to advise medical personnel of the best ways of overcoming the "cultural peculiarities" presumably inhibiting the target population's "acceptance" of modern health care. Rather, to paraphrase Alan Beals (1979:690), it should be to insure that the community has genuinely available its fair share of whatever medical services its government is capable of providing.

EVALUATING THE APPROACH

Decisions that Pichatareños make about treatment come about through an interaction of two kinds of influences. The first derive from the culturally patterned knowledge about illness and its treatment that residents have in mind in making treatment choices. The second are a product of the real world conditions within which people make these choices, but over which they have little direct control in specific illness situations—particularly those conditions determining the accessibility of nonindigenous treatment alternatives. To explain meaningfully the distribution of treatment choices in a community requires that the role of each kind of influence be made clear.

If we fail to distinguish carefully between these influences, we run the risk of attributing certain choices to one kind of influence when they are in fact due in much greater degree to the other. As I reviewed above, for example, this appears to be the case in Pichatáro for choices that seem primarily influenced by real world constraints (such as high costs in relation to available resources) but which might be explained instead as primarily influenced by traditional illness beliefs and attitudes. Of course, the disparity in the policy implications of the two sets of findings is great.

If we employ the decision-making approach the likelihood of such errors is lower than with the correlational approach characteristic of much previous research on medical choice (see Chapter One). This is because with a correlational approach the explanation that is ultimately reached is as much dependent upon the specific variables the investigator chooses to examine as it is upon the actual factors involved in people's choices. If we collect data solely on the acculturative status of the individuals using different treatment alternatives, for example, then the explanation for their differential utilization will necessarily be cast in these terms. With the decision-making approach, on the other hand, nothing about the method of investigation determines the ultimate content or form of the model; it is free to reflect whatever combination of factors actually determines a given community's choices.

The decision-making approach that has been followed here represents a relatively recent development in the area of cognitive anthropology, a line of research that was at one time characterized as a "science of trivia" (Harris 1968:591). It seems fair to say, on the basis of the results of this study and of the limited number of other applications of the decision-making approach (see Chapter One), that we have good evidence to the contrary. Our approach has not only provided detailed insights into an issue that is, by most standards, significant, but it has also made explicit the relationship between the ideational and the observable in a way that would seem difficult to accomplish by other means.

Presenting one's research findings in anthropology is really never anything more than a progress report. The determinants of human behavior can never be known or described with certainty, and each set of findings leads in turn to a new set of questions that require answers. In the present case there are several such questions.

Future research should be directed toward further examining the cognitive bases of the treatment decision-making process. As I have discussed in more detail elsewhere (Young 1980), the dynamics of the faith concept, in particular, remain incompletely known. Faith, as I have described it in this study, has at least two aspects—as a judgment of the relative likelihood of cure associated with each system of therapy, and as a generalized likelihood of cure ranking associated with each treatment alternative. Only further field research can clarify the exact nature and range of information considered in such judgments, and the relationship between situational faith judgments and the more generalized rank ordering.

Another issue that this study puts us in a good position to examine in the future is change in the treatment decision-making process itself. As I mentioned in Chapter One, variation in the observable patterning of health-care choices through time does not necessarily indicate change in the underlying standards by which people make these choices. Because we have some understanding of this underlying process, it should be possible to determine whether future shifts in the utilization of modern medical services represent true culture change (as ideational change; see Goodenough 1963:269) or just a relaxation of external accessibility constraints on these choices.

Finally, future study should examine some of the extracommunity determinants of treatment decisions. It is clear that much of what determines the nature of health care and medical choice in Pichátaro derives from the community's marginal position in relation to the national society. Because this study has focused on medical choice from the point of view of the individual seeking treatment, it has been possible only to touch upon the larger external political and economic realities. It is these, however, that will ultimately determine whether health care in Pichátaro will improve.

By pursuing these questions, perhaps some day we shall come to understand even more fully the ways in which the people of Pichátaro continue—as they so often say—to "make the struggle" against illness.

Appendixes

A

Case Collection Procedures

To provide case history materials for use in testing the model of treatment decision making, we selected sixty-two Pichátaro households to visit on an approximate biweekly basis during a six-month period in 1976. We again surveyed the households during a return visit in June through August 1977. In all, 323 illness episodes were recorded.

THE SAMPLE

Originally, we randomly selected a sample of fifty-two households (approximately 10% of the town) from the town census. Each household was then visited, the project explained, and permission asked to make regular visits over the following few months. All households contacted agreed to participate. After the first two rounds of visits, however, we decided to replace five of the households, as they were uncooperative (a child was always sent to the gate to report that "no one" was home—an acceptable strategy in Pichátaro when one wishes not to be disturbed), and it seemed likely that we would be unable to get an accurate record of illness occurrences from them. We selected replacements by searching the census sheets for other households that matched the originals as closely as possible in terms of size, *barrio* membership, occupation, language use, education, and so on. Later it became necessary to replace two more households (the families had gone to Mexico City), and this was done in the same manner.

After the first round of case collection visits, we decided to add an additional ten households to the sample, randomly selected from the *barrio* of San Miguel. This was done in order to increase the number of cases obtained from the upper part of town (see Chapter Two), with the idea of later comparing certain aspects of illness behavior between the two parts. No significant differences were found, however, and the cases have therefore been combined with those obtained from the original sample of fifty-two households.

Although the sample is not a strictly random one, it does represent the town in terms of mean household size, occupation, education, language use, house type, and so on. We can assume that the body of data collected is also representative of Pichátaro households in general.

CASE COLLECTION PROCEDURES

Each household in the sample was visited on an approximate biweekly schedule. The actual time between visits varied from about ten to fifteen days, dependent upon whether return visits were necessary, and upon how much other interviewing was being done at the same time. At each visit an adult member of the household was questioned. In cases where no adults were at home, up to two return visits were made before a given household was skipped for that round. Visits were begun in February of 1976, and continued until late July—a period just short of six months. At each visit, household members were questioned about any illnesses that had occurred since the previous visit. If illnesses had been recorded during the last visit, we also collected information on their progress or resolution.

The intent of the case collection was to record all illnesses in each household during the six-month survey period. Especially in the early rounds, we urged informants repeatedly during the visit to report all illnesses that had occurred, no matter how minor. We kept an account of each illness on a specially prepared form, on which its entire course could be charted in detail. Figure A.1 illustrates how one of the cases described in Chapter Six (Enrique's first case of *gripa*) was recorded. We kept records on a day-by-day basis of symptoms present, their severity, the cause ascribed to the illness, the treatment actions taken, behavioral changes accompanying the illness, and the family's reaction. Any changes as the illness

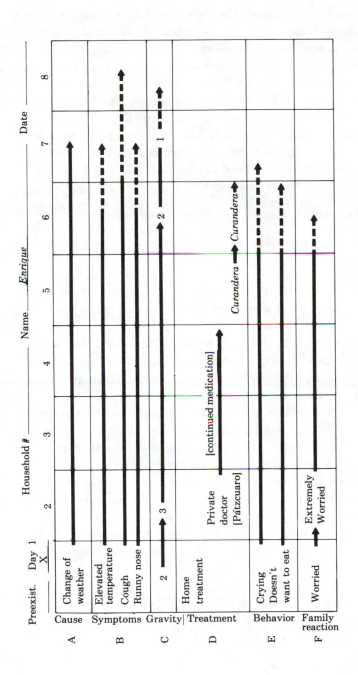

Figure A.1. **Enrique's Case of *gripa***

progressed could be indicated.[1] (In the actual field interviewing, the symptoms, treatments, causes, and so on, were coded and recorded by number.) Elsewhere on the form we entered the diagnostic label(s) given the illness episode, and additional information on the treatment alternatives utilized (their cost and location, the outcome of the treatment, and so on). Once the details of the illness were obtained, we discussed the case less formally and asked the informant about the situation that led up to the choice of treatment, why other alternatives had not been chosen, and what further actions were being considered in the event that the illness continued. We thus made the attempt to get as much information as possible concerning the reasoning behind the choice of treatment.

ADDITIONAL DATA ON THE
SAMPLE HOUSEHOLDS

In addition to the information available from the general town census for each sample household, we collected three other types of data.

Wealth rankings were obtained for each household. We asked five key informants to rank the households on their relative level of wealth (according to their *recursos económicos*). The actual task involved sorting a set of cards, one for each *jefe de familia* ('household head') in the sample, into an unspecified number of groups, depending on the wealth differences judged to exist between them. Informants formed from six to nine groups. Overall, agreement between raters was high,[2] and there was little difficulty in performing the task. Raters were chosen from various parts of town for their special knowledge of these matters (for example, one was a storekeeper, one worked in the tax collector's office). These ratings were combined and an overall wealth rank assigned to each household. The ranks were put to several uses in the analysis (see Chapter Six).

The other two areas in which we collected supplementary data are the family illness histories discussed in Chapter Six ("Testing the Model" section) and the socioeconomic data in Appendix B.

B

A Correlational Analysis

By the correlational approach I refer to studies which have posited single factors or classes of related factors as explaining
differential treatment choices, because of their association with
them.[1] As discussed in Chapter One, the basic explanation emerg-
ing from such studies is most often one of the following: 1. different
categories of people use different treatment sources because they
have different beliefs or expectations about their effectiveness, and
therefore treatment choices are predictable on the basis of the acculturative status, educational background, or some other specified
feature of the informant;[2] or 2. people believe a given type of treatment or practitioner capable of curing only specific classes of illness, and therefore treatment choices are predictable on the basis of
the characteristics of the illness involved.

In order to test how well such factors relate to different treatment choices in the Pichátaro data, I compiled the following characteristics of the sample households: educational level and literacy
of both male and female household heads; educational attainment
of their children; age of the male household head; language use
(Tarascan and Spanish); media exposure (radio and television
ownership, and newspaper and magazine reading habits); frequency of travel outside of Pichátaro; migratory experience in
other areas of Mexico; migratory experience in the United States;
the relative wealth rank of the household; and the primary occupation of the male household head. In addition, I constructed two
composite variables—one an education variable combining the
schooling, literacy, language use, and media exposure items; the
other an outside exposure variable combining travel and migration.
I also compiled a second set of factors dealing with illness episodes:
category of illness (derived from the analysis in Chapter Four);

etiological category; level of gravity; duration of the illness; and the age, sex, and birth order of the victim of the illness.

I then determined the statistical association of each of these factors with the treatment choices in the illness cases described in Chapter Six. These cases were placed into five groups according to the treatment alternative(s) used in each: 1. those receiving only home or self-treatment; 2. those taken to a folk curer; 3. those taken to a *practicante;* 4. those taken to a physician (private physician or the Pátzcuaro Health Center); and 5. those in which both a folk curer and a physician were consulted. Cases were placed in categories 2 through 5 regardless of whether they received prior self-treatment. Eighty-four percent of the cases could be placed in the above categories; the remaining 16% involved a wide variety of treatment combinations, none of which was frequent enough to be included as a separate category. Since these latter cases do not together form a homogeneous group, I excluded them from the present analysis. I then constructed a series of twenty-two contingency tables. In each case, the five treatment categories served as the dependent variable, and each of the factors described in the preceding paragraph served, in turn, as the independent variable. The aim was to see how well the independent variables predicted the distribution of the cases across the different treatment categories.

For each table, I computed a measure of statistical significance (chi square) and two measures of strength of association (Cramer's *V* and lambda). Nine of the factors were significantly associated (significance level for chi square of less than .05) with the treatment choices. These are listed in Table B.1, along with their corresponding values for *V* and lambda. Since at least one variable (the treatment categories) in each case is at the nominal level, more frequently encountered measures of association such as Pearson's *r* and Spearman's rho are not appropriate. Cramer's *V*, a measure of association for two nominal-level variables, is simply the phi statistic adjusted for tables larger than 2×2, and like phi its value ranges from zero to $+1$. I also calculated a second measure of association, lambda, since it provides a convenient interpretation: it represents (in its asymmetrical form) the percentage by which ability to predict the dependent variable (the treatment choices) is im-

Table B.1.   **Factors Associated with Treatment Choices**

Factor	Significance level for χ^2	V	Lambda	
			Asym.	Sym.
Wealth rank of household	0.0001	0.29	0.04	0.07
Occupational type	0.001	0.20	0.00	0.00
Education of children	0.0001	0.21	0.00	0.06
Media exposure	0.01	0.20	0.00	0.05
Illness category	0.0001	0.27	0.03	0.06
Etiological category	0.0001	0.23	0.00	0.03
Level of gravity	0.0001	0.58	0.24	0.29
Duration of illness	0.0001	0.31	0.09	0.07
Age of victim	0.0001	0.24	0.00	0.07

proved once knowledge of the independent variable (each of the nine factors in Table B.1) is provided. The symmetrical form of lambda, also included, measures overall predictive improvement when no assumptions are made about which variable is independent. (For additional discussion of V and lambda, see Blalock 1972:295–303; Mueller et al. 1970:249–256; and Nie et al. 1975: 224–226.)

If we examine the results, it is apparent that no single factor by itself substantially accounts for the overall distribution of treatment choices. Many of the factors in the table are not independent of each other. Educational attainment of children and media exposure, for example, are both significantly and positively correlated with wealth. Similarly, the age of the victim and the duration of the illness are both important considerations in judging the gravity of an illness (see Chapter Three). Thus, in many cases the factors are not independent predictors of treatment choices.

Some conclusions, however, are possible on the basis of these results. The highest association occurs with the level of illness gravity, which alone improves the rate of prediction by 24%. One can reasonably infer, then, that the gravity of an illness is an important factor influencing treatment choices. It is also apparent that relative household wealth is influential.[3] On the whole, the results compare favorably with those obtained in other studies of this type. Colson's (1971) data from a rural Malay village, for example, show a V value (my computation) of 0.53 for the relationship between severity and choice of treatment, which is quite close to that obtained here. He demonstrates a slightly higher association ($V = 0.54$) with illness etiology, however, contrary to what I found for these data. Gould (1965) also claims a relationship between illness severity/incapacitation and choices of indigenous versus scientific therapy in a village in India, although it is unclear in what way the actual data presented support his hypothesis. DeWalt (1977), in examining the relationship of different sociodemographic factors to the use of a single alternative (physicians) in a rural Mexican village, found that to explain just over half of the variance in use, six different variables had to be entered into the regression equation. In general, then, the present results do not appear greatly different from those obtained in other studies of the correlational type. They therefore provide at least an approximate reference point for comparison with the success rate of the decision model tested in Chapter Six.

C

Representing the Data on Treatment Choice

The principal task in analyzing the paired comparisons and other treatment decision data was to determine the ways in which the main considerations involved combined in a given instance and led to the selection of a particular treatment alternative. Since, owing to the nature of the data, fragments of these utilization rules are scattered across many responses, it was necessary to combine them and eliminate redundancies. What I sought, then, was a means of formalizing the narrative descriptions of treatment choice that were available from the interviews. Two possible means by which this may be accomplished are flow charting the data or using a decision table.

Flow charts are frequently used to describe decision processes (see C. Gladwin 1975; Geoghegan 1973; Keesing 1971). Figure C.1 illustrates how the following narrative can be charted:

> There are two reasons why people here go to curers. When the sickness is not grave and they think that the curer can cure it, they go to her. Or, if the sickness is grave and they lack the money to go to a doctor they go to her.

An alternative means of formalizing narratives is the decision table. Decision tables specify: 1. the conditions (considerations) affecting choices; 2. the actions that may be taken; and 3. the rules of choice, that is, the particular combinations of conditions that lead to each action. The methodology behind the use and construction of decision tables is well developed (Pollack et al. 1971; see also Miller and Johnson-Laird 1976:281–290). The sample narrative may be put in decision-table format as shown in Table C.1.

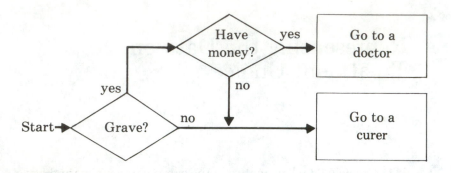

Figure C.1.   **Flow Chart of Narrative**

The Y's ("yes") in the table indicate that the particular condition must be true or present for that rule; the N's ("no") indicate that the condition must be false or absent. A blank indicates that the condition is not relevant for that rule—that it may take any value and not affect the action taken. Criteria for a good table are that it cover all possible combinations of conditions (completeness), and that each combination be covered only once (nonredundancy). In the example below, since there are two conditions, each of which may take two values, there are (2×2) or four possible combinations, or rules. However, since Rule 3 covers two combinations, namely $(\overset{N}{N})$ and $(\overset{N}{Y})$, the table is complete. Conditions are not nec-

Table C.1.   **Model Decision Table**

Rules	*1*	*2*	*3*
Conditions			
Grave	Y	Y	N
Have money	Y	N	
Actions			
Go to a doctor	x		
Go to a curer		x	x

essarily limited to binary values. For example, rather than "yes" and "no" for Condition 1, the entries might have been slightly, moderately, and very grave, had the narrative contained these distinctions. In this case the condition would have three possible values, and the table six possible rules.

Both flow charts and decision tables contain the same information, and one may readily translate from one to the other, as has just been shown. For present purposes, I have found the decision table to provide the clearer and more straightforward format for formalizing the data on choice of treatment. As the number of conditions to be considered increases, the drafting task involved in constructing a flow chart becomes more complex, and the chart is less easily read than the equivalent decision table. One might argue that the decision table ignores the ordering of considerations (assessments) and that the flow chart preserves this order. All that is actually lost, however, is the impression of the temporal order of consideration of conditions, and not their logical order or priorities (H. Gladwin 1975:188). In the narrative gravity has priority over having money, since the latter is a relevant consideration only in cases of grave illness. Gravity, on the other hand, is relevant in all situations. The flow chart could be redrawn with "have money" in the first diamond; a "no" for that condition would lead directly to the choice of a curer. This is not the ordering of considerations expressed in the narrative, however, and so this representation would be inaccurate. It is of course not difficult to detect such errors in this example, but in more complex cases involving more considerations and choices among more alternatives, mistakes are less easily avoided. Reversing the ordering of conditions in the decision table, on the other hand, would result in no difference in how the rules are defined, and the logical ordering or priorities of the conditions would remain.

Note that the decision table does not describe what is involved in the determination that, for example, a given illness is indeed grave or that one does have money sufficient for a visit to a doctor. These matters are discussed in the text.

Notes

CHAPTER ONE

1. A number of contrasting terms are used in the literature to distinguish the more localized systems of medical belief and practice that characterize particular cultural traditions from scientifically based biomedicine. Here, the former will be referred to as traditional, folk, indigenous, or non-Western, and the latter as modern, Western, or scientific.

2. While not reviewed here, the sociologically oriented literature on health care utilization is quite extensive and may be consulted by those interested in additional approaches (see Andersen, et al. 1975; Anderson 1973).

3. The sample queries that Janzen provides (1978:33), however, are not exemplary of ethnoscience interviewing techniques.

4. Other examples of the "features of the illness" approach include Chen 1975; Colson 1971; Gould 1965; and Logan 1973. A few studies have examined treatment choices with reference to features of both the illness and the people, for example, Cosminsky 1972; Garrison 1977.

5. I prefer "account for" rather than "predict," since the test data usually represent choices that have already been made.

6. Apart from the question of convenience (we were both already fluent in Spanish), other factors suggested that the use of Spanish as the primary field language was appropriate. The majority of Pichátaro's adults are bilingual (Tarascan and Spanish); of those that are not, nearly all are monolingual Spanish speakers. It became reasonably clear to us early in the fieldwork that Spanish was as much the language of illness as was Tarascan. In inquiring about illness terminology in Tarascan, for example, many times informants were unable to recall a term, finally responding: "I don't remember the Tarascan word for it, but here it's called _____" (using a Spanish term). We learned only enough Tarascan to amuse people with our attempts to speak it.

7. This number includes forty-five cases collected from the same sample of households during the return trip in 1977.

CHAPTER TWO

1. Additional ethnographic details on Pichátaro, and a fuller presentation of the quantitative data referred to in this chapter, may be found in Young (1978b).

2. "San Francisco" refers to the town's patron saint, and for some purposes forms a part of the town's official name. Ordinarily it is referred to simply as Pichátaro.

3. The Tarascan region includes two other areas as well—la Cañada, on the northern boundary of the Sierra, and the area around Zacapu—which are not described here because of their distance from, and lesser importance for, Pichátaro. An excellent geographic summary of the Tarascan region may be found in West (1948), from which many of the details included in this paragraph were taken.

4. No attempt will be made here to review the substantial ethnographic literature on the Tarascan area. R. Beals (1969) references most of the important sources up to about 1960. Castile (1972:44–46) reviews several works which appeared during the 1960's. See also the studies of Acheson 1972a, b; Burgos Guevara 1964; Dinerman 1974, 1978; G. Foster 1967.

5. All Pichátaro forest lands are communally owned, and household heads are assigned certain sections for such purposes as firewood and resin collection. These "holdings" may be neither bought nor sold.

6. This contrasts with the situation in the neighboring village of Cumachuén. During a visit there, several men with whom we spoke lamented the town's critical land shortage, which was responsible for many leaving to seek work in Zamora and Mexico City.

7. This is in great contrast to what Foster claims for Tzintzuntzan, in the Lake area. These people, when asked about wealth differences, are said to characteristically respond "There are no wealthy men, here we are all equal!" (G. Foster 1967:12).

8. The use to which these data were put becomes apparent in Chapter Six.

9. Although most agricultural lands in Pichátaro are officially communal property, individuals have rights to the use of particular parcels. Such parcels are frequently bought and sold within Pichátaro, and while such transactions have no legal basis in state law, they are recognized within the town itself.

10. Households in Pichátaro form small "corporations" (Hunt and Nash 1967) since taxes and assessments for special community events, such

as the major fiestas, are levied on a household rather than on an individual basis.

11. This is a brief ceremony in which the crown of a saint's image is placed momentarily on the child's head to insure his or her proper healthy growth.

12. San Bartolo I has an abandoned chapel that houses no saint's image. In 1977 attempts were underway to renovate the structure. One can see badly preserved ruins of the chapel of San Francisco. In the other *barrios*, older people can remember the former locations of their respective chapels, but the sites are now occupied by houses.

13. See G. Foster (1960:34) and Kearney (1972:22–24) for further discussion of the upper-lower phenomenon in other Mesoamerican communities.

14. Fortunately, and purely by chance, our house in Pichátaro was very near the fuzzy line separating the upper and lower parts of town, and thus carried no strong identification with either (see Figure 2.2 for this boundary's location.)

15. Many details on governmental organization in the Tarascan area may be found in Moone (1969).

16. There is a good deal of support in Pichátaro for the idea of becoming a separate *municipio,* a status which will be quite difficult to achieve.

17. Sometimes referred to as the *representante de bienes comunales* ("Representative of Communal Properties").

18. Van Zantwijk (1967:209) lists a number of ceremonial offices Pichátaro "has," which were actually abandoned many years ago. His use of the ethnographic present seriously confounds the comparisons he attempts; for example, the source of his comments on Pichátaro is Leon's (1904) nineteenth-century work in the area. In this connection, see Carrasco (1952).

CHAPTER THREE

1. This sensation is apparently produced by throbbing of the aorta.

2. The symptoms of *latido* seem closely akin to what Western medicine terms an "anxiety reaction," a type of neurosis (see Butcher 1971:25–27). Clark (1959:178–179) describes the same illness in a Mexican-American community in California.

3. One woman disagreed, saying that women must be more resistant than men, since they must be able to withstand their husbands' blows!

4. Water is considered essential in preventing the body from drying out, but no informant was able to provide details of its utilization. It is simply drunk to "take away the thirst," collected in the *bazo,* passed to the bladder (if this is distinguished from the *bazo*), and eliminated.

5. Cosminsky's (1975, 1977a) description of the concept *alimento* in a Guatemalan community is in some ways parallel to what we described for Pichátaro, although in this case there is apparently no equation of juiciness with strength.

6. This should not be confused with the wet-dry dichotomy of classical humoral theory (see G. Foster 1953), to which the present juicy-dry distinction appears unrelated. Whereas "wetness" and "dryness" in the humoral scheme were not necessarily related to actual moisture content (W. Madsen 1955), what is specifically of concern here is the water or oil content of the food.

7. "Hot" or "cold" in quotes refers to an item's supposed quality (as with foods); without the quotes, to actual temperatures.

8. He refers to two American nurses who have operated a clinic for some years in this lake village. They are renowned in the area for their fluency in Tarascan.

9. For additional discussion of the concept of contagion, see Chapter Four, note 7.

10. Chapter Four explores how this awareness is reflected in illness categorization.

11. Conditions involving spots on the skin approximating those produced by smallpox are usually designated in Pichátaro as *viruela loca* ('crazy smallpox'), considered to be a distinct, less serious form of smallpox.

12. Data on the number of alternatives used per episode are given in Chapter Six.

13. The average rank-order correlation (Spearman's rho) between informants on the illness term ranking task was 0.46, as compared with 0.55 for the symptom rankings.

14. Two symptoms—*calentura* (a "temperature") and *tos* ('cough')—are not indicated in Table 3.1, for reasons discussed below.

15. However, informants rarely disagreed by greater than one level.

16. "Bed" is used loosely here, since many Pichatareños sleep on simple woven mats rather than in beds.

17. The other symptom remaining unclassified was *tos* ('cough'). This is because different kinds of coughs are recognized ('dry cough,' 'rasping cough'), and they indicate varying levels of gravity.

18. In the sorting task, the symptom "vomiting" was explained as referring to a severe type that we might associate with, say, acute dysentery.

CHAPTER FOUR

1. This technique and several other features of the study reported in this chapter are adapted from D'Andrade, et al. (1972), and are similar in several respects to procedures discussed in Kronenfeld and Kronenfeld (n.d.).

2. The decision to set the cutoff at six or more was made after examination of the frequency distribution of the number of "yeses" per frame-term pair across the ten informants, which showed an inflection at five. The mean number of "yeses" received by frame-term pairs recorded affirmatively in the data matrix is 7.3; for those recorded as "no" the mean number is 1.7. Overall, then, the data matrix reflects a greater than 70% consensus. Raising the cutoff point to, say, seven or more would have eliminated over one-fifth of the positive cases in the data matrix, while increasing the average consensus only 4%.

3. There are no set rules for the selection of a similarity measure for cluster analysis. The principal issue in this case is whether or not negative matches (both items lack the given attribute) should be included. In the course of the analysis similarity measures were calculated in both ways, and the clusterings done on them were quite similar. The differences that did occur would not substantially change the conclusions here. For a number of frames elimination of negative matches would disregard a significant attribute. For example, that two illnesses are both not grave illnesses is fully as significant as the fact that two others are. In my reckoning about one-third of the frames are of this type. For other frames negative cases seem less significant (for example, two illnesses both do *not* give you chills) but still cannot be considered irrelevant. With these considerations in mind I decided to include both positive and negative matches in the similarity figures. Another possibility in the calculation of a similarity measure is to assign greater weight to certain attributes that are thought for intuitive or theoretical reasons to have greater importance. However, in this case I was interested in examining the categories that result in the absence of assumptions about the significance of particular distinctions, so I did not attempt to weight the attributes.

4. The Johnson clustering procedure actually produces two representations of the data. Initially it takes the two most similar items and joins them. This cluster is then linked to the item most similar to it to form a second cluster, and so on. Were the data perfectly hierarchical, items merged would have the same similarity profile, but in practice this is rarely the case. Johnson's first solution, the "connectedness" method, uses the distance between an item and the member of the cluster most similar to it as its measure of the similarity of an item to the cluster. His "diameter" method takes the distance of an item to the member of the cluster least similar to it as its measure. Miller (1969:190–191) points out that for each of these solutions there is a matrix corresponding to the levels at which each pair of items clusters. Construction of this matrix consists of tracing up from each pair of items to the point at which they were first included in the same cluster. The matrices corresponding to both the connectedness and the diameter solutions for the present data were constructed and correlated (Spearman rank-order correlations) with the original similarities data. The results were: original-connectedness = 0.70; original-diameter = 0.74. The diameter representation was therefore selected, on the basis that it provided the better fit with the original data, and is the representation given in Figures 4.1 and 4.2.

5. The term and the general idea come from Bruner, Goodnow, and Austin (1956, Chap. 2), although I have devised the specific application. Note that criteriality is not a measure of statistical association. It seems closely analogous to what some cognitive psychologists refer to as "cue validity" (see Rosch 1978). Calculation of criteriality values is not limited to cases in which cluster analysis has been used, but is generally applicable in situations where a classification of items, and information on the distribution of a set of characteristics across those items, are available.

6. One might wonder if the removal of low variance frames discussed a few pages earlier resulted in the elimination of any additional highly criterial attributes. The distribution of these attributes across clusters was checked, and none had a significant criteriality. The main effect of including low variance frames in the data is to increase the similarity levels overall, with little influence on the resulting clusters.

7. The local understanding on contagion bears no strong resemblance to the germ theory. It can be shown that a relationship exists between the attribute *hot weather* and the attribute *contagion* (see Figure 4.5). Logically, possession of the attribute *contagion* implies possession of

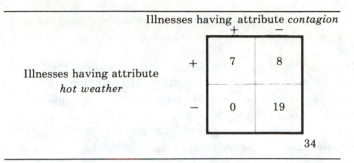

Figure 4.5.   **Relationship between Hot Weather and Contagion**

the attribute *hot weather,* since there is no case of an illness having the former while lacking the latter. On the basis of the ethnographic evidence, one may infer a causal relation between the two, hot weather being a necessary, but not sufficient, condition of contagion (see D'Andrade 1976). For the illnesses in cluster I (Figure 4.1) hot weather is believed to make a person more susceptible to "attacks" of cold from an air or moisture and thus may be viewed as a condition predisposing one to certain illnesses stemming from contact with external environmental hazards. The relationship between hot weather and the illnesses having this attribute in cluster II is that heat generated from within the body, as from work or strong emotions, is not readily dissipated as it would be in the more temperate weather existing during most of the year.

8. This distinction also seems to have been made in classical Greek and Roman medicine, to which Latin American ethnomedicine is historically related (G. Foster 1953). The Greek physician Galen wrote concerning sources of deterioration:

> But since [the body] has two sources of deterioration, one intrinsic and spontaneous, the other extrinsic and accidental, it must needs require no little care and forethought. Now it has been shown that intrinsically the body first deteriorates and declines toward death in two ways, either from old age or from the perpetual flux of its substance, or, as a consequence of what it eats and drinks, from the formation of excrements. Spontaneously, then, it thus deteriorates. But of those things which affect it from without, certainly one which is inseparable and, as we might say, essential is the surrounding atmosphere

. . . [which] harms us by making us unduly warm or cold, dry or moist. . . . (Green 1951:11).

9. The distinction proposed by G. Foster (1976) between "personalistic" and "naturalistic" causality concepts involves a different sort of consideration. He refers primarily to the extent to which volitional agents are implicated in explaining illness. Here, however, the reference to personal illnesses is meant only to establish that the initiating circumstances are conceived as internal to the individual.

CHAPTER FIVE

1. Home and self-treatment are used here interchangeably; both refer to situations in which the ill person either treats himself or is treated by another household member, and no curing specialist is consulted or otherwise involved.
2. Until recently it was common for Tarascans to refer to themselves ethnically as *naturales* or *naturalitos* ('natural people'), contrasting with *gente de razón* ('people of reason') or mestizos (see Chapter Two).
3. Neither was he referred to as a *huesero* ('bonesetter') or *sobador* ('masseuse'), which are specialized curing roles common in some areas of Mexico (see Adams and Rubel 1967).
4. One might then question employing use of traditional curers as an index of commitment to traditional beliefs, as is sometimes done in modernization studies employing a correlational design.
5. This was also true at the time of Beals's study of Cherán (R. Beals 1946:156–158).
6. "Center of Fundamental Education for Community Development in Latin America," a UNESCO and Organization of American States sponsored training center in Pátzcuaro.
7. To avoid the confusion that might result from using the English translation for this category of curing specialists, the Spanish *practicante* will be used, with the understanding that it refers specifically to this particular type of "practitioner." Note that this is not the more usual meaning of the term, which generally denotes graduates of medical schools who are practicing prior to their receiving formal certification as physicians.
8. In general, men report fewer illnesses than women, but not to the extent of accounting for the difference discussed here.
9. The medical school curriculum in Mexico consists of five years.

10. One woman referred to the nurses working at the Center as *criadas* ('maids')!

11. In Mexico most drugs legally requiring a doctor's prescription for their sale may in fact be bought without one in many pharmacies.

12. This view has some justification. See Cañedo (1974) for documentation of the overwhelmingly urban concentration of health care personnel and facilities in Mexico. The Ario de Rosales Clinic represents some attempt on the part of the Mexican Government to alleviate this maldistribution.

13. Most Pichátaro residents, along with rural subsistence farmers generally in Mexico, do not receive regular wages nor belong to organizations that would permit enrollment in the Social Security system and thus are excluded from using the regular I.M.S.S. Clinics found in most towns and cities (see the discussion of institutionalized exclusion in Chapter Two).

14. Simoni and Ball (1975) present an interesting discussion of marketplace medicine hucksters. Their observations were made in several locations in Mexico, including the Pátzcuaro market.

CHAPTER SIX

1. It was claimed (in Chapter One) that the decision-making approach offers a number of potential advantages, particularly compared with the correlational approach. The evaluation of this claim requires that some consideration also be given to the results that the latter approach yields in accounting for the same data. Such an analysis is described in Appendix B.

2. This is not always the case. Quinn (1976), for example, describes the difficulties involved in eliciting explanations of how pacification fees are set in Mfantse litigation proceedings. In the present case, however, our success in obtaining the decision criteria seems to have been largely due, in addition to the importance and recurrence of such decisions, to the fact that people are used to talking about them.

3. The case histories mentioned here are not those which were briefly summarized at the beginning of this chapter (and at the end of Chapter Three). The latter constitute a separate body of cases from an entirely different sample of Pichátaro households, and their primary use is as test cases for the model developed later in this chapter.

4. The reason that the two now-excluded alternatives were included initially was that the interviews were begun early in the fieldwork period,

before any of the case history data, and much of the data in Chapter Five, were available.

5. By juxtaposing folk and medical treatment, as is frequently done in this chapter, I do not mean to suggest that folk treatment is not medical in the broad ethnographic sense of the term. I simply chose these as the best translations of the terms Pichatareños use to refer to the two systems of therapy and to avoid more cumbersome terms (such as "folk medical treatment" and "Western scientific-based medical treatment").

6. The figures in Table 6.3 reflect the percentage of equivalent responses for each pair of hypothetical situations across all informants. For a given pair, each instance in which two informants stated that the same alternative would be used at the same stage in the sequence of treatment was counted as one "agreement." The figures were arrived at as follows:

$$\frac{\text{number of agreements} - \text{number of disagreements}}{\text{total possible agreements}}.$$

Therefore, positive figures in Table 6.3 indicate that agreements outnumber disagreements, while negative figures indicate that disagreements outnumber agreements. The figure itself indicates the magnitude of the difference. For example, in pair (3, 4) agreements outnumber disagreements by 68% of the total responses, which means that of all responses, 84% (that is, $.68 + (1.0 - .68)/2$) were in agreement.

7. Note that two figures are given for some of the pairs in Table 6.3. These are the pairs of situations that are the same except for the last consideration—knowledge of a remedy. When a remedy is known, it is almost always described as the first step that would be taken. Therefore, for these situations, when the informant is subsequently asked what would next be done assuming the remedy had been ineffective, the situations are now the same: a remedy is not known in either case. The second figure given in these cases is the agreement between the two sets of responses when the initial "known remedy" step is eliminated. In some cases (such as 1, 2) the responses are very similar; in others (such as 5, 8), the difference in initial conditions seems to have considerable effect in reducing the subsequent similarity of the responses.

8. A note on terminology: "considerations" and "conditions" both refer to the four criteria identified in the paired comparison interviews, and subsequently incorporated into the model. When cited as particular components of the model, they are called "conditions"; in other contexts it seems more appropriate to refer to them as "considerations."

9. The contrast between the two processes just described is analogous to what are referred to in the literature on decision making as "marking rules" and "assessments," respectively (see Geoghegan 1973; Quinn 1974).

10. Actually faith has been spoken of in this section in two somewhat different ways—as the situationally variable judgment of the relative likelihood of cure associated with each system of therapy (folk and Western medical) just described, and as a generalized likelihood of cure ranking associated with each treatment alternative (as in Figure 6.1). However, *within* each system of therapy the ranking of alternatives is generally fixed: if one judges medical treatment as more likely to provide a cure, a physician's treatment will, on this aspect, be ranked over a *practicante,* and a *practicante* over self-treatment; if one estimates folk treatment as more likely, that provided by a curer will be ranked over that provided by self-treatment. This is why when a faith judgment is necessary, the basis upon which it is made is the system of therapy. Once judged, the relative ordering of individual alternatives involving the class of therapy is fixed. Note that all the faith concept implies is an ordinal estimate of relative probabilities ($prob_a > prob_b$) and not the construction of a probability distribution (as in, for example, Fabrega's [1974:169–174] illness behavior model), the cognitive plausibility of which is questionable (see Quinn 1978; Young 1980:125–127).

11. The reason for this is that the type of medical remedies available for home treatment are not considered as "strong" as those used by *practicantes;* the remedies used by curers, on the other hand, are not greatly different from those used in home treatment.

12. Note that the faith condition never involves a tautology, since a given value (F or M) does not in itself indicate an unambiguous choice (F may lead to either self-treatment or a curer, and M to any except a curer). Faith in folk treatment, for example, is a necessary but not sufficient condition for the choice of a folk curer.

13. In the course of testing, eighteen choices were eliminated because they involved treatment alternatives not included in the model, and

twenty-seven were eliminated because insufficient data were obtained to score them reliable.

CHAPTER SEVEN

1. The most extreme and blatantly ethnocentric expression of this point of view that I have encountered is contained in Schendel's *Medicine in Mexico*:

> At the very bottom of the cultural scale are the isolated, pure-blooded tribes of indigenes, who dwell in remote areas unreached by missionaries or any other aspects of modern civilization. In such "pockets of history," some literally still live in the Stone Age. Speaking only their ancient tribal language, they retain their traditional pagan beliefs and customs 100 percent. . . . Among these people, belief in old Indian deities, evil spirits, and the powers of sorcery is, naturally, absolute. And the witch doctor provides the only "medical" attention available. . . . This belief in evil powers as an important cause of illness sends the ignorant flocking to *curanderos* and *brujos* for treatment, rather than to doctors of medicine (Schendel 1968:134–135).

2. This particular example was chosen for citation because the implications for policy have been made particularly explicit. It is not difficult to find similar explanations from studies made a good deal closer to Pichátaro. Woods, for example, in regard to modern health-care utilization in a Guatemalan community, concludes that "the persistence of the Indian's traditional world view is perhaps the most pervasive reason for Luceño reluctance to relinquish use of their folk practitioners" (Woods 1977:44).

3. Here is how the rejected alternatives were determined: take Rule 6.4–2 of the model (Table 6.4) as our first example. The illness is initially judged as nonserious, thus, by the cost-ordered strategy assumed in effect, a physician's treatment would not be an option under consideration. Further, self-treatment has been considered and eliminated, as no home remedy is known in this case. It may reasonably be assumed, then, that the actor at this point is left to choose between a curer and a *practicante*, and thus the choice of a curer may be said to most directly entail the rejection of a *practicante*'s treatment. Rule 6.4–7, on the

other hand, defines a situation of grave illness, in which a probability-of-cure ordered strategy would be in effect. Since no other condition is specified that would eliminate the choice of a physician (such as inaccessibility) except the faith consideration, the choice of a curer here may be said to most directly entail the rejection of a physician's treatment. Since the choice process involves rank orderings of alternatives along particular dimensions (see Figure 6.1), it is generally the case that for each specific choice another alternative may be designated as the second most plausible option to have been chosen, and thus also as that most directly rejected.

4. As I pointed out in Chapter Two, Pichátaro is less poor and less isolated than many rural indigenous communities in Mesoamerica, whose disadvantage in terms of health care is proportionally even greater.

APPENDIX A

1. The method of recording the illnesses is adopted from Fabrega (1974:185–189). The case collection procedures in general parallel those used by Colson (1971), and Woods and Graves (1973).
2. The Kendall coefficient of concordance (W) for the five sets of ratings was 0.77 (significant at the 0.001 level) (see Siegel 1956:229–238).

APPENDIX B

1. Examples are cited in Chapter One.
2. Surprisingly, the possibility that some alternatives are used more frequently by those who can best afford them has been given less attention.
3. As will be seen later in Chapter Six, there are good reasons why these particular items should do this well.

Glossary

Only Spanish terms used repeatedly are included here. Terms are defined as they are used in the context of illness in Pichátaro.

aire   An "air" or "wind," usually a "cold" agent that may cause illness by entering the body and upsetting its normal "hot"-"cold" equilibrium.

bilis   The "gall bladder," an internal body part containing a dangerous liquid that may be released and spread through the body as a result of strong emotional experiences. Also, the name for the illness so brought about. The term *hiel* is usually taken as synonymous with *bilis*.

brujo   A "witch," who may be sought for the cure (and presumably at times the "causation") of witchcraft-related illnesses. Also referred to as an *hechicero*. This term does not generally refer to folk medical practitioners *(curanderas)*.

buena enfermedad   "Good illness," i.e., brought about through natural means rather than through witchcraft. Contrasts with *mala enfermedad*.

calentura   A state of elevated temperature or bodily "heat," which accompanies many illnesses. Also used as a diagnostic label for conditions in which elevated temperature is the only significant symptom. *Calentura* is not synonymous with *fiebre* ("fever"), since the latter refers to a specific, severe state of excessive bodily heat.

caseros   See *remedios caseros*.

comadre   Between a child's parents and godparents, the female term of reference and address.

compadrazgo   The enduring, kinlike, ritually formed relationship linking parents and godparents.

compadre   Between a child's parents and godparents, the male term of reference and address.

curandera(o)   "Curer," a traditional or folk curing specialist. Often referred to simply as "one who knows [how to cure]." In Pichátaro, curers are almost always women.

descuido   "Carelessness." Illnesses thought brought about by contact with an external environmental hazard are often attributed to *descuido*, the implication being that the victim bears some responsibility for the illness.

209

enfermedad   "Illness" or "sickness."

fe "Faith" or "confidence." As a consideration in the treatment decision-making process, *fe* refers to a subjective judgment of the relative likelihood of cure associated with folk, versus modern, treatment and remedies in curing the given type of illness.

fuerza   "Strength" or "vigor." Obtained from food and air, *fuerza* is the basis of bodily functioning. Most body parts may be explained in terms of their role in the provision, distribution, or utilization of *fuerza*.

gripa   "Cold" or "flu," the most common illness in Pichátaro.

latido   "Pulsating ball," literally "palpitation." A body part described as a small ball located behind the navel, which may "rise up" and cause illness in response to eating delays. Also, the name for the resulting illness.

mal de ojo   "Evil eye." An illness specific to children, thought caused by someone's strong emotional reaction after seeing a child. This reaction is somehow transferred to the child, causing one of two types of illness: if the child has "light" blood, *ojo de gusto* ("of delight") will result; if the child has "dark" blood, *ojo de coraje* ("of anger"), a much more serious illness, will result. This illness is thought curable only through folk treatment methods.

mala enfermedad   "Bad" or "evil" illness, thought to be caused by witchcraft. (Contrasts with *buena enfermedad*.)

médico   A physician.

médicos   See *remedios médicos*.

mollera caída   "Fallen fontanel," an illness, usually confined to children, thought to result when a section of the top of the skull "falls down" as a result of a fall or fright. This illness is considered curable only through folk treatment methods.

ojo   See *mal de ojo*.

practicante   Literally, a "practitioner," but in Pichátaro used to refer specifically to nonphysician practitioners of modern medicine, either the local Catholic nuns (who run a small dispensary), a government-employed nurse, or a local self-trained lay "doctor."

remedios caseros   "Folk remedies" (literally, "household remedies"). Refers to the herbal and other plant- and animal-derived medicinal substances used in traditional illness treatment. Used both in self-treatment and by folk curers.

remedios médicos   "Medical remedies" or "doctors' remedies." Refers to both pharmaceuticals and manufactured patent medicines. *Remedios médicos* are associated with physicians and *practicantes*, and remedies classified as such may also be used in self-treatment.

References

Acheson, James M.
 1972a Limited Good or Limited Goods? American Anthropologist
   74:1152–1169.
 1972b Accounting Concepts and Economic Opportunities in a Tarascan
   Village: Emic and Etic Views. Human Organization 31:83–91.
Adams, Richard N.
 1952 Un análisis de las creencias y prácticas médicas en un pueblo
   indígena de Guatemala. Instituto Indigenista Nacional, Publica-
   ciones Especiales, no. 17. Guatemala.
 1974 Harnessing Technological Development. In Rethinking Modernization. John J. Poggie, Jr., and Robert N. Lynch, eds. pp. 37–68.
   Westport, Conn.: Greenwood Press.
Adams, Richard N., and Arthur J. Rubel
 1967 Sickness and Social Relations. In Social Anthropology. Manning
   Nash, ed. pp. 333–356. Handbook of Middle American Indians,
   vol. 6. Robert Wauchope, gen. ed. Austin: University of Texas
   Press.
Aguirre Beltrán, Gonzalo
 1967 Regiones de refugio. Instituto Indigenista Interamericano, Edi-
   ciones Especiales 46. Mexico, D.F.: Instituto Indigenista Inter-
   americano.
Anderberg, Michael R.
 1973 Cluster Analysis for Applications. New York: Academic Press.
Andersen, Ronald, Joanna Kravits, and Odin W. Anderson
 1975 Equity in Health Services: Empirical Analyses in Social Policy.
   Cambridge, Mass.: Ballinger.
Anderson, James G.
 1973 Health Service Utilization: Framework and Review. Health Services Research 3:184–199.
Barkin, David
 1975 Regional Development and Interregional Equity: A Mexican
   Case Study. In Latin American Urban Research, vol. 5. Wayne A.
   Cornelius and Felicity M. Trueblood, eds. pp. 277–299. Beverly
   Hills, Calif.: Sage Publications.

Barth, Fredrik
   1967   On the Study of Social Change. American Anthropologist 69:661–
           669.
Beals, Alan R.
   1976   Strategies of Resort to Curers in South India. *In* Asian Medical
           Systems. Charles Leslie, ed. pp. 184–200. Berkeley: University of
           California Press.
   1979   *Review of* Anthropology in the Development Process, Hari
           Mohan Mathur, ed. American Anthropologist 81:689–690.
Beals, Ralph
   1946   Cherán: A Sierra Tarascan Village. Smithsonian Institution, In-
           stitute of Social Anthropology, publication no. 2. Washington,
           D.C.: U.S. Government Printing Office.
   1969   The Tarascans. *In* Ethnology, p. 2. Evon Vogt, ed. pp. 725–773.
           Handbook of Middle American Indians, vol. 8. Robert Wauchope,
           gen. ed. Austin: University of Texas Press.
Benyoussef, Amor, and Albert F. Wessen
   1974   Utilization of Health Services in Developing Countries—Tunisia.
           Social Science and Medicine 8:287–304.
Blalock, Hubert M., Jr.
   1972   Social Statistics, 2d ed. New York: McGraw-Hill.
Brown, Cecil H.
   1976   General Principles of Human Anatomical Partonomy and Specu-
           lations on the Growth of Partonomic Nomenclature. American
           Ethnologist 3:400–424.
Brown, Cecil H., et al.
   1976   Some General Principles of Biological and Non-Biological Folk
           Classification. American Ethnologist 3:73–85.
Bruner, Jerome S., Jacqueline J. Goodnow, and George A. Austin
   1956   A Study of Thinking. New York: John Wiley.
Burgos Guevara, Hugo
   1964   Medicina campesina en transición. Thesis, Escuela Nacional de
           Antropología e Historia, Mexico, D.F.
Burton, Michael
   1972   Semantic Dimensions of Occupation Names. *In* Multidimen-
           sional Scaling, vol. 2: Applications. A. Kimball Romney, Roger N.
           Shepard, and Sara Beth Nerlove, eds. pp. 55–71. New York: Semi-
           nar Press.
Butcher, James N.
   1971   Abnormal Psychology. Belmont, Calif.: Brooks/Cole.

Cañedo, Luis
    1974   Rural Health Care in Mexico? Science 85:1131–1137.

Carrasco, Pedro
    1952   Tarascan Folk Religion. Tulane University, Middle American Research Institute, publication no. 17.

Castile, George P.
    1972   Cherán: The Adaptation of an Autonomous Community in Michoacán, Mexico. Ph.D. dissertation, Anthropology Department, University of Arizona.

Chen, Paul C. Y.
    1975   Medical Systems in Malaysia: Cultural Bases and Differential Use. Social Science and Medicine 9:171–180.

Clark, Margaret
    1959   Health in the Mexican-American Culture. Berkeley: University of California Press.

Colson, Anthony
    1971   The Differential Use of Medical Resources in Developing Countries. Journal of Health and Social Behavior 12:226–237.

Cosminsky, Sheila
    1972   Utilization of a Health Clinic in a Guatemalan Community. Atti del XL Congreso Internazionale degli Americanisti, Roma-Genova, pp. 329–338. Genoa: Tilgher.
    1975   Changing Food and Medical Beliefs and Practices in a Guatemalan Community. Ecology of Food and Nutrition 4:183–191.
    1977a Alimento and Fresco: Nutritional Concepts and Their Implications for Health Care. Human Organization 36:203–206.
    1977b The Impact of Methods on the Analysis of Illness Concepts in a Guatemalan Community. Social Science and Medicine 11:325–332.

Craine, Eugene R., and Reginald Reindorp, eds. and trans.
    1970   The Chronicles of Michoacán. Norman: University of Oklahoma Press.

Currier, Richard L.
    1966   The Hot-Cold Syndrome and Symbolic Balance in Mexican and Spanish-American Folk Medicine. Ethnology 5:251–263.

D'Andrade, Roy G.
    1976   A Propositional Analysis of U.S. American Beliefs about Illness. *In* Meaning in Anthropology. Keith H. Basso and Henry A. Selby, eds. pp. 155–180. Albuquerque: University of New Mexico Press.

D'Andrade, Roy G., Naomi Quinn, Sara Beth Nerlove, and A. Kimball Romney

1972   Categories of Disease in American-English and Mexican-Spanish. *In* Multidimensional Scaling, vol. 2: Applications. A. Kimball Romney, Roger N. Shepard, and Sara Beth Nerlove, eds. pp. 9–54. New York: Seminar Press.

DeWalt, Kathleen M.

1977   The Illnesses No Longer Understand: Changing Concepts of Health and Curing in a Rural Mexican Community. Medical Anthropology Newsletter 8(2):5–11.

Dinerman, Ina

1974   Los tarascos. SepSetentas no. 129. Mexico, D.F.: Secretaría de Educación Pública.

1978   Economic Alliances in a Mexican Regional Economy. Ethnology 17:53–64.

Douglas, Bill G.

1969   Illness and Curing in Santiago Atitlán. Ph.D. dissertation, Anthropology Department, Stanford University.

Dunn, Fred L.

1976   Traditional Asian Medicine and Cosmopolitan Medicine as Adaptive Systems. *In* Asian Medical Systems, Charles Leslie, ed. pp. 133–158. Berkeley: University of California Press.

Erasmus, Charles J.

1952   Changing Folk Beliefs and the Relativity of Empirical Knowledge. Southwestern Journal of Anthropology 8:411–428.

1961   Man Takes Control. Minneapolis: University of Minnesota Press.

Ewald, Robert

1967   Directed Change. *In* Social Anthropology. Manning Nash, ed. pp. 490–511. Handbook of Middle American Indians, vol. 6. Robert Wauchope, gen. ed. Austin: University of Texas Press.

Fabrega, Horacio, Jr.

1972   Medical Anthropology. *In* Biennial Review of Anthropology, 1971, Bernard J. Siegel, ed. pp. 167–229. Stanford: Stanford University Press.

1974   Disease and Social Behavior. Cambridge: MIT Press.

Firth, Raymond

1951   Elements of Social Organization. London: Watts.

Fisher, Lawrence E., and Oswald Werner

1978   Explaining Explanation: Tension in American Anthropology. Journal of Anthropological Research 34:194–218.

Fjellman, Stephen

1976   Natural and Unnatural Decision-Making: A Critique of Decision Theory. Ethos 4:73–94.

Foster, George M.
  1953   Relationships between Spanish and Spanish-American Folk Medicine. Journal of American Folklore 66:201–217.
  1958   Problems in Intercultural Health Practice. Pamphlet no. 12. New York: Social Science Research Council.
  1960   Culture and Conquest: America's Spanish Heritage. Viking Fund Publications in Anthropology, no. 27.
  1967   Tzintzuntzan: Mexican Peasants in a Changing World. Prospect Heights, IL: Waveland Press.
  1976   Disease Etiologies in Non-Western Medical Systems. American Anthropologist 78:773–782.
  1979   Methodological Problems in the Study of Intracultural Variation: The Hot/Cold Dichotomy in Tzintzuntzan. Human Organization 38:179–183.
Foster, George M., and Barbara Gallatin Anderson
  1978   Medical Anthropology. New York: Wiley.
Foster, Mary L.
  1969   The Tarascan Language. University of California Publications in Linguistics, vol. 56.
Frake, Charles O.
  1961   The Diagnosis of Disease Among the Subanun of Mindanao. American Anthropologist 63:113–132.
Friedrich, Paul
  1969   On the Meaning of the Tarascan Suffixes of Space. International Journal of American Linguistics (part 2) 35(4):1–48.
  1970   Agrarian Revolt in a Mexican Village. Englewood Cliffs, N.J.: Prentice-Hall.
  1976   A Phonology of Tarascan. University of Chicago Studies in Anthropology, no. 4.
Garrison, Vivian
  1977   Doctor, Espiritista or Psychiatrist?: Health-Seeking Behavior in a Puerto Rican Neighborhood of New York City. Medical Anthropology 1(2):66–191.
Geertz, Clifford
  1973   Thick Description: Toward an Interpretive Theory of Culture. *In his* The Interpretation of Cultures pp. 3–30. New York: Basic Books.
Geoghegan, William
  1973   Natural Information Processing Rules: Formal Theory and Applications to Ethnography. Monographs of the Language-

Behavior Research Laboratory, no. 3. Berkeley: University of California Language-Behavior Research Laboratory.

Gladwin, Christina H.

1975   A Model of the Supply of Smoked Fish from Cape Coast to Kumasi. *In* Formal Methods in Economic Anthropology. Stuart Plattner, ed. pp. 71–127. Special publication of the American Anthropological Association, no. 4. Washington, D.C.: American Anthropological Association.

1976   A View of the Plan Puebla: An Application of Hierarchical Decision Models. American Journal of Agricultural Economics 58:881–887.

1977   A Model of Farmers' Decisions to Adopt the Recommendations of Plan Puebla. Ph.D. dissertation, Food Research Institute, Stanford University.

Gladwin, Hugh

n.d.   Limitations of Verbal Eliciting Techniques in Providing a Model of Decision Making. Manuscript.

1975   Looking for an Aggregate Additive Model in Data from a Hierarchical Decision Process. *In* Formal Methods in Economic Anthropology. Stuart Plattner, ed. pp. 159–196. Special publication of the American Anthropological Association, no. 4. Washington, D.C.: American Anthropological Association.

Gladwin, Hugh, Michael Murtaugh, and Christina H. Gladwin

1978   Understanding Understanding Decision Making. Manuscript, School of Social Sciences, University of California, Irvine.

Goodenough, Ward H.

1956   Residence Rules. Southwestern Journal of Anthropology 12:22–37.

1963   Cooperation in Change. New York: Russell Sage Foundation.

1964   Introduction. *In* Explorations in Cultural Anthropology. W. H. Goodenough, ed. pp. 1–24. New York: McGraw-Hill.

Gould, Harold

1965   Modern Medicine and Folk Cognition in Rural India. Human Organization 24:201–208.

Green, Robert M., trans.

1951   A Translation of Galen's Hygiene. Springfield, Ill.: Charles C. Thomas.

Harris, Marvin

1968   The Rise of Anthropological Theory. New York: Crowell.

Harwood, Alan
  1971   The Hot-Cold Theory of Disease. Journal of the American Medical Association 216:1153–1158.
Holland, William R.
  1963   Medicina maya en los altos de chiapas. Mexico, D.F.: Instituto Nacional Indigenista.
Hunt, Eva, and June Nash
  1967   Local and Territorial Units. *In* Social Anthropology. Manning Nash, ed. pp. 253–282. Handbook of Middle American Indians, vol. 6. Robert Wauchope, gen. ed. Austin: University of Texas Press.
Ingham, John M.
  1970   On Mexican Folk Medicine. American Anthropologist 72:76–87.
Janzen, John M.
  1978   The Quest for Therapy in Lower Zaire. Berkeley: University of California Press.
Johnson, Stephen C.
  1967   Hierarchical Clustering Schemes. Psychometrika 32:241–254.
Kay, Paul
  1970   Some Theoretical Implications of Ethnographic Semantics. *In* Current Directions in Anthropology. Ann Fischer, ed. pp. 19–31. Washington, D.C.: American Anthropological Association.
Kearney, Michael
  1972   The Winds of Ixtepeji. New York: Holt, Rinehart and Winston.
  1977   Oral Performance by Mexican Spiritualists in Possession Trance. Journal of Latin American Lore 3:309–328.
Keesing, Roger M.
  1971   Formalization and the Construction of Ethnographies. *In* Explorations in Mathematical Anthropology. Paul Kay, ed. pp. 36–49. Cambridge: MIT Press.
Kronenfeld, David B., and Jerrold E. Kronenfeld
  n.d.   What a Fanti Needs to Know in Order to Treat a Kinsman Correctly. Paper delivered at the Mathematical Social Sciences Board Advanced Research Seminar in Natural Decision-Making, Palo Alto, California, December 13–17, 1971.
León, Nicolas
  1904   Los tarascos. Notas históricas, étnicas y antropológicas. 3 vols. Mexico, D.F.: Museo Nacional de México.
Leslie, Charles, ed.
  1976   Asian Medical Systems. Berkeley: University of California Press.

Logan, Michael
   1973   Humoral Medicine in Guatemala and Peasant Acceptance of
           Modern Medicine. Human Organization 32:385–395.
Madsen, Claudia
   1965   A Study of Change in Mexican Folk Medicine. Tulane University,
           Middle American Research Institute, publication 25.
Madsen, William
   1955   Hot and Cold in the Universe of San Francisco Tecospa, Valley of
           Mexico. Journal of American Folklore 68:123–129.
Maloney, Clarence, ed.
   1976   The Evil Eye. New York: Columbia University Press.
Margolies, Barbara Luise
   1975   Princes of the Earth. Special publication of the American An-
           thropological Association, no. 2. Washington, D.C.: American An-
           thropological Association.
Matras, Judah
   1973   Populations and Societies. Englewood Cliffs, N.J.: Prentice-Hall.
McClain, Carol
   1977   Adaptation in Health Behavior: Modern and Traditional Medi-
           cine in a West Mexican Community. Social Science and Medicine
           11:341–347.
Metzger, Duane, and Gerald Williams
   1963   A Formal Ethnographic Analysis of Tenejapa Ladino Weddings.
           American Anthropologist 65:1076–1101.
Mexico
   1963   Octavo censo general de población: Estado de Michoacán. Mex-
           ico, D.F.: Secretaría de Indústria y Comercio, Dirección General
           de Estadística.
Miller, George A.
   1969   A Psychological Method to Investigate Verbal Concepts. Journal
           of Mathematical Psychology 6:169–191.
Miller, George A., and Philip Johnson-Laird
   1976   Language and Perception. Cambridge: Belknap.
Mintz, Sidney W. and Eric Wolf
   1950   An Analysis of Ritual Co-Parenthood (Compadrazgo). South-
           western Journal of Anthropology 6:341–368.
Moerman, Daniel E.
   1974   Extended Family and Popular Medicine on St. Helena Island,
           S.C.: Adaptations to Marginality. Ph.D. dissertation, Anthropol-
           ogy Department, University of Michigan.

Molony, Carol H.
  1975   Systematic Valence Coding of Mexican "Hot"-"Cold" Food. Ecology of Food and Nutrition 4:67–74.

Moone, Janet
  1969   Tarascan Development: National Integration in Western Mexico. Ph.D. dissertation, Anthropology Department, University of Arizona.

Mueller, John, Karl Schuessler, and Herbert Costner
  1970   Statistical Reasoning in Sociology, 2d ed. Boston: Houghton Mifflin.

Nash, June
  1967   The Logic of Behavior: Curing in a Maya Indian Town. Human Organization 26:132–140.

Nie, Norman H., et al.
  1975   Statistical Package for the Social Sciences, 2d ed. New York: McGraw-Hill.

Parsons, Talcott
  1951   The Social System. Glencoe, Ill.: The Free Press.

Pollack, Solomon L., Harry T. Hicks, Jr., and William J. Harrison
  1971   Decision Tables: Theory and Practice. New York: Wiley.

Press, Irwin
  1969   Urban Illness: Physicians, Curers and Dual Use in Bogotá. Journal of Health and Social Behavior 10:209–218.

Quinn, Naomi
  1974   Getting Inside Our Informants' Heads. Reviews in Anthropology 1:244–252.

  1975   Decision Models of Social Structure. American Ethnologist 2:19–45.

  1976   A Natural System Used in Mfantse Litigation Settlement. American Ethnologist 3:331–351.

  1978   Do Mfantse Fish Sellers Estimate Probabilities in Their Heads? American Ethnologist 5:206–226.

Ravicz, Robert
  1967   Compradrinazgo. *In* Social Anthropology. Manning Nash, ed. pp. 238–252. Handbook of Middle American Indians, vol. 6. Robert Wauchope, gen. ed. Austin: University of Texas Press.

Rosch, Eleanor
  1978   Principles of Categorization. *In* Cognition and Categorization. Eleanor Rosch and Barbara B. Lloyd, eds. pp. 27–48. Hillsdale, N.J.: Lawrence Erlbaum Associates.

Schendel, Gordon
    1968   Medicine in Mexico: From Aztec Herbs to Betatrons. Austin: University of Texas Press.
Schwartz, Lola
    1969   The Hierarchy of Resort in Curative Practices: The Admiralty Islands, Melanesia. Journal of Health and Social Behavior 10:201–209.
Siegel, Sidney
    1956   Nonparametric Statistics for the Behavioral Sciences. New York: McGraw-Hill.
Simmons, Ozzie G.
    1955   Popular and Modern Medicine in Mestizo Communities of Coastal Peru and Chile. Journal of American Folklore 68:57–71.
Simon, Herbert A.
    1957   Models of Man: Social and Rational. New York: Wiley.
Simoni, Joseph J., and Richard A. Ball
    1975   Can We Learn from Medicine Hucksters? Journal of Communication 25:174–181.
Swadesh, Mauricio
    1969   Elementos del tarasco antiguo. Mexico, D.F.: Universidad Nacional Autónoma de México.
Turner, Victor
    1968   Drums of Affliction. Oxford: Clarendon Press.
Tversky, Amos
    1972   Elimination by Aspects: A Theory of Choice. Psychological Review 79:281–299.
Tversky, Amos, and Daniel Kahneman
    1974   Judgment Under Uncertainty: Heuristics and Biases. Science 185:1124–1131.
Tyler, Stephen A., ed.
    1969   Cognitive Anthropology. New York: Holt, Rinehart and Winston.
Valentine, Charles A.
    1968   Culture and Poverty: Critique and Counterproposals. Chicago: University of Chicago Press.
van Zantwijk, Rudolf
    1967   Servants of the Saints. Assen, The Netherlands: Van Gorcum.
Wallace, Anthony F.C.
    1970   Culture and Personality, 2d ed. New York: Random House.
Werner, David
    1975   Donde no hay doctor, 2d ed. Mexico, D.F.: Impresora Galve.

West, Robert C.
  1948 Cultural Geography of the Modern Tarascan Area. Smithsonian Institution, Institute of Social Anthropology, publication no. 7. Washington, D.C.: U.S. Government Printing Office.

White, Douglas R.
  1973 Mathematical Anthropology. *In* Handbook of Social and Cultural Anthropology. John J. Honigmann, ed. pp. 369–446. Chicago: Rand-McNally.

Whitten, Norman E., Jr., and John F. Szwed
  1970 *Introduction to* Afro-American Anthropology. Norman E. Whitten, Jr., and John F. Szwed, eds. pp. 23–60. New York: The Free Press.

Woods, Clyde M.
  1977 Alternative Curing Strategies in a Changing Medical Situation. Medical Anthropology 1(3):25–54.

Woods, Clyde, and Theodore D. Graves
  1973 The Process of Medical Change in a Highland Guatemalan Town. Latin American Studies Series, vol. 21. Los Angeles: University of California Latin American Center.

Young, James C.
  1978a Illness Categories and Action Strategies in a Tarascan Town. American Ethnologist 5:81–97.
  1978b Health Care in Pichátaro: Medical Decision Making in a Tarascan Town of Michoacán, Mexico. Ph.D. dissertation, Anthropology Department, University of California, Riverside.
  1979a Variation in a Mexican Folk Medical Belief System. Paper presented at the annual meetings of the Southern Anthropological Society, Memphis, Tenn., Feb.
  1979b *Review of* The Evil Eye, Clarence Maloney, ed. Medical Anthropology Newsletter 10(3):19–20.
  1980 A Model of Illness Treatment Decisions in a Tarascan Town. American Ethnologist 7:106–131.

Index